# EFFECTIVE WAYS TO LOWER YOUR ODDS OF GETTING CANCER

# EVERYDAY CANCER RISKS AND HOW TO AVOID THEM

EFFECTIVE WAYS TO LOWER
YOUR ODDS OF GETTING CANCER

# EVERYDAY CANCER RISKS AND HOW TO AVOID THEM

## MARY KERNEY LEVENSTEIN

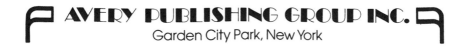
AVERY PUBLISHING GROUP INC.
Garden City Park, New York

Cover Design: Janine Eisner-Wall and Rudy Shur
In-House Editor: Marie Caratozzolo
Typesetter: Bonnie Freid
Photo Credits: Adrienne Burack
Original Artwork: Ann Vestal

Dedication page exerpt has been reprinted with permission.

**"THE WIND BENEATH MY WINGS"**
(Jeff Silbar, Larry Henley)
©1982 WB GOLD MUSIC CORP. and
WARNER HOUSE OF MUSIC
All Rights Reserved. Used By Permission.

**Library of Congress Cataloging-in-Publication Data**

Levenstein, Mary Kerney.
    Everyday cancer risks and how to avoid them : effective ways
to lower your odds of getting cancer / Mary Kerney Levenstein.
    p. cm.
    Includes bibliographical references and index.
    ISBN 0-89529-505-9

    1. Cancer—Prevention. 2. Cancer—Risk factors. I. Title.

RC268.L48  1992                                    92-18103
616.99'405—dc20                                    CIP

Printed in the United States of America

10  9  8  7  6  5  4  3  2  1

# CONTENTS

*For Earle*

*Did you ever know that you're my hero?*
*You're everything I would like to be.*
*I can fly higher than an eagle*
*For you are the wind beneath my wings.*

# ACKNOWLEDGMENTS

For their support when I was diagnosed with cancer and throughout my surgery and treatment—the experience that inspired this book—I acknowledge with thanks and love:

My husband, Earle, for the nights he spent sleeping on a chair next to my hospital bed, for an inner strength that carried me when my own strength wavered, and for a love that transcends the limits of this lifetime.

My daughter Cairistin, for grieving with me, celebrating with me, and believing with me that I could make a difference in my own healing process.

My daughter Ruth, for encouraging me with her gentle spirit and reassuring me with her faith in God and in life as a loving teacher.

My stepdaughter, Cathy, for keeping me surrounded with love and healing consciousness.

My mother, Elsie Kerney, for her example of serenity, courage, and healing from within.

My sister, Ellen Kerney, for making room for my fears and listening to them.

My brother Regan Kerney, for knowing how hard it was and for bolstering my determination with his own resolution and resilience.

My brother Lincoln Kerney, for bringing the great gift of laughter back into my heart when I thought I had only tears inside.

Ann Erdman, for lighting the way through some dark summer nights.

Toni Pew, for taking such loving care of my children.

Nancy Ticktin, for constancy and caring over so many years.

Cordelia Biddle, for being there when I returned from surgery and for sharing the full spectrum of my feelings.

Johnny B. Clontz, for showing me that it is possible to become stronger in the broken places.

Howard Miller, for teaching me that stumbling blocks can be transformed into opportunities.

Isadore From, for listening and for helping me find solace and fortitude within.

Jim Burke, for his Peruvian tale of la Cellita's Inca spirit.

My agent and dear friend, Mary Yost, for her largeheartedness, grace, and inspiration.

Maria Tucci Gottlieb, for her compassionate presence the day I was diagnosed, for bringing bagels to the hospital every morning, and for leading me to Julie Winter.

My therapist and teacher, Julie Winter, for being an instrument of healing love, spiritual guidance, and deep wisdom.

\* \* \*

For their support throughout the research and writing of this book, I acknowledge with thanks and everlasting appreciation:

My publisher, Rudy Shur, for his broad vision and his belief in me.

My editor, Marie Caratozzolo, for her insights, guidance, and help in ensuring the clarity and accuracy of this book.

The many colleagues and organizations that responded promptly and thoroughly, again and again, to my queries; especially the staffs of the American Cancer Society, the Centers for Disease Control, the Childhood Cancer Institute, Citizens Clearinghouse for Hazardous Waste, the Community Nutrition Institute, the Center for Science in the Public Interest, the Food and Drug Administration, Food and Water, Inc., the Environmental Defense Fund, the Environmental Protection Agency, the National Agricultural Library, the National Cancer Institute, the National Coalition Against the Misuse of Pesticides, the Natural Resources Defense Council, the Nuclear Information and Resource Service, the Radioactive Waste Campaign, the United States Department of Health and Human Services, and the United States Public Information Research Group.

# FOREWORD

Most people in America and around the world fear cancer because it is associated with a feeling of hopelessness and a painful and slow death. Currently, one of every three Americans will develop cancer and by the year 2000, two of every five.

Despite the declaration of war on cancer in 1971 by President Nixon, and the consequent investment of billions of dollars for research, the number of new cases and the number of deaths from cancer rise every year. About $75 billion is spent on cancer treatment yearly. New treatments are often trumpeted by scientists and the news media, most fizzle out quickly.

From 1930 to 1992—despite the introduction of radiation therapy, chemotherapy, and immunotherapy; despite CT scans, MRI scans, and all the other new medical technology— lifespans for almost every form of cancer have remained the same, which means only one thing—there has been no significant *progress* in the treatment of cancer. And worse yet, perhaps even consistent with deception, is the unrealistic goal set by the National Cancer Institute and the American Cancer Society of a 50 percent reduction in cancer mortality by the year 2000. I have been convinced that this goal could never be attained because of the almost vertical rise in new cancer cases each year. And late in 1991, the Government Accounting Office, an independent agency, determined the same—there has been no progress in the treatment of cancer, with very few exceptions (some of the children's cancers). Because of this, we must turn our attention to prevention.

After reviewing the existing cancer data, I found that 80–90 percent of all cancers develop from lifestyle choices we make and substances to which we are exposed. For instance, 60 percent of women's cancers and 40 percent of men's cancers are related to nutritional factors alone; 30 percent of all cancers are related to tobacco exposure. We must: modify our diets and take certain nutrients; avoid tobacco altogether; minimize or eliminate alcohol; avoid unnecessary radiation; insist that the environment is clean; avoid sexual promiscuity, hormone use, and unnecessary drugs; learn the early warnings of cancer; exercise more; and learn how to relax, have fun, and have better interpersonal relationships. These are all simple preventive measures.

Mary Kerney Levenstein's simple-to-read book, *Everyday Cancer Risks and How to Avoid Them,* outlines many risk factors for developing cancer and then explains what you can do about each one. A major asset of the book is it provides names, addresses, and oftentimes, toll-free numbers of concerned groups or agencies, which you can call to explore these issues.

It is your responsibility to learn of and then modify your own risk factors in order to prevent cancer and heart disease. You, your family, and particularly your children will benefit enormously. The earlier in life a prevention plan is initiated, the healthier a person will be. Giving a *healthy start* to young children will keep them well and ultimately produce a healthy society. The cost for health care will eventually dwindle. Levenstein's book should be part of your anti-cancer plan.

You have almost total control over the destiny of your health. Seize this opportunity!

Charles B. Simone, M.MS., M.D.
Founder and Director of
Simone Cancer and Immunology Center
Author of *Cancer and Nutrition*

# PREFACE

Having cancer changed my life completely. The quality of my life today is immeasurably better than it was before I had cancer, and for that reason I never look back and wish that cancer hadn't happened to me. On the contrary, I see that it was a very special gift. It helped me learn to live each day fully, with mindfulness of being and a deep sense of inner peace. While I would recommend other, less stressful routes to this level of self-actualization, the fact is that my path lay through cancer, and without it, I would not be where I am today.

My memories of being diagnosed with cancer are crisp and vivid. I can still see the pained look on the surgeon's face as he told me that the lump in my breast was malignant. I remember how stricken my husband, Earle, looked when he heard the news. I can see myself sitting perfectly still on the edge of the examining table, watching, listening, hearing Earle and the surgeon talk, and thinking how strange it was that they seemed to be moving and speaking in slow motion.

As I sat there, another conversation was going on in my head. "Cancer. Does this mean that I'm going to die soon? What about my children? Will I live to see Cairistin and Ruth have children of their own? What do I know about cancer? Aren't there are a lot of people who have survived cancer? If there is even one person who has survived, it means that I have a chance. I don't know any survivors, I don't know who they are, but I'm going to find out. I'm going to find out how they did it, and I'm going to survive too."

From that very moment I began to immerse myself in the cancer experience. The next day, three days before my surgery, Earle and I went out to look for books and tapes on healing. I began listening to deep-relaxation and meditation tapes. I read every book I could find on surviving cancer. I learned that doctors Carl Simonton, a radiation oncologist, Bernie Siegel, a surgeon, and Lawrence LeShan, a clinical psychologist, were using a variety of healing techniques with cancer patients. I contacted them to find out what resources they could recommend for me.

I arranged for a consultation with Dr. LeShan, who urged me to begin experiencing more of my own inner ecology, to mobilize all the healing and self-healing techniques available, and to recognize and fulfill my own dreams. Earle and I went to a workshop given by Dr. Siegel, where we began to understand that, with a positive attitude, cancer can be met as a challenge and turned into an opportunity for growth and change. I began to use Dr. Simonton's visual-imagery techniques to reduce stress, to affirm my expectations of a successful outcome, and to enhance my own immune system function. I started working with Julie Winter, a psychotherapist whose work incorporates a healing consciousness. I began to examine the stress issues and the unresolved conflicts in my life. I began to pray. And I began to heal.

I was learning a lot about spiritual and emotional healing, but, naturally, I was also looking for a healing process for my body. After all, that was where the cancer had shown up. One day, I was astonished to read that the United States Department of Health and Human Services estimated that 80 percent of cancer is related to lifestyle, to choices that most of us can freely make. I wanted to know exactly what I could do to reduce these risks.

I started gathering data from federal agencies, from consumer health and environmental organizations, from medical libraries, and from research institutions. I soon realized that, in fact, *very few* things cause cancer, and that most are within our reach to do something about.

I began eating differently, gradually adopting a high-fiber, low-fat, additive-free vegetarian diet. I increased my exercise time to one hour, six times a week. I had a water filter installed in our home, and asked people not to smoke in our house. Bathroom and kitchen shelves were emptied of products that contained hazardous ingredients and were refilled with non-toxic alternatives. I installed a radiation shield on my computer monitor screen, and I tested our ceramic dishes and bowls to be certain that they were not leaching lead. Our house was tested for radon. We committed ourselves to recycling our household paper, aluminum, and glass; we built a compost pile for food and yard wastes; and we discovered that a local hazardous-waste collection site accepted dead batteries and other toxic items. (In the process, we reduced our garbage volume by 95 percent.) Earle not only supported me but also joined me in all my efforts. Soon I began to feel that my eating habits, my home, my environment, and my lifestyle were truly healthy.

Initially, I felt great frustration at not being able to find a comprehensive source of information on the everyday risks of cancer in my life. Most important, I wanted information on what I could do about these risks. As I began to gather facts, I became a resource for my friends and neighbors. I ultimately decided that the best way to share what I had learned was to put all this information together in one book.

According to current statistics, one out of every three people in the United States is expected to get cancer; over the years, it will affect three out of four families. I hope this book will help you begin to make the choices and changes that remove you from these statistics. These choices and changes can lead not only to an improvement in your own personal health but also to a healthier world in which we and the generations that follow us can live.

# INTRODUCTION

Most people are confused about what does and does not cause cancer. Often, the reaction to this uncertainty is a feeling of being out of control. The easy way out is to conclude that everything causes cancer, so why fight it. It's easier to throw up one's hands in resignation and give up. But there's no need to feel overwhelmed. Everything *doesn't* cause cancer. The good news is that you can avoid a significant number of cancers by simply changing some of your habits. You have the power to reduce cancer risks dramatically, even if there is a history of cancer in your family. You live in a world filled with pollution, chemicals, artificial ingredients, and stress, but you can make a commitment to change your own little corner of it, and a lot of little corners add up to significant change.

The United States Department of Health and Human Services estimates that approximately 80 percent of human cancer is related to lifestyle—to such aspects of daily life as the food you eat, the air you breathe, the places you live and work, your stress response, and whether or not you smoke or exercise. According to current statistics, one out of every three people in this country will get cancer in their lifetime; over the years, three of every four families will be affected. But by changing even a few habits, you can turn these odds around and greatly increase your chances of being one of those who will not develop cancer. The single most effective way to fight cancer is to prevent it.

Cancer has been with us throughout history. It was found in dinosaur fossils as well as in mummies of South America and ancient Egypt. Recent statistics are provided in Table 1. This table presents the 1991 mortality rates due to cancer for every state in the United States (in descending order). Given are the actual cancer deaths per 100,000 people, and the total number of deaths in 1991 compared with the total number of newly diagnosed cases that year.

Some carcinogens initiate cancer directly by changing normal cells into cancerous cells. Other carcinogens promote cancer indirectly by fostering opportunistic conditions for cancer to develop. When combined, many carcinogens interact to produce an exponentially higher cancer risk than each separate agent would produce alone. For instance, an American Cancer Society study showed that smokers who are exposed to asbestos increase their risk of lung cancer by as much as 90 times, or 9,000 percent.

**Table 1    Estimated U.S. Cancer Statistics, 1991**

| State | Death Rate per 100,000 | Number of Deaths | Number of New Cases |
|---|---|---|---|
| 1. District of Columbia | 222 | 1,700 | 3,600 |
| 2. Maryland | 194 | 9,800 | 21,000 |
| 3. Delaware | 190 | 1,400 | 3,100 |
| 4. Alaska | 189 | 500 | 1,200 |
| 5. Louisiana | 187 | 9,000 | 19,100 |
| 6. Nevada | 185 | 2,300 | 4,900 |
| 7. New Jersey | 185 | 18,400 | 39,100 |
| 8. Virginia | 182 | 12,100 | 26,000 |
| 9. Ohio | 182 | 24,300 | 52,000 |
| 10. Kentucky | 181 | 8,100 | 17,300 |
| 11. Rhode Island | 181 | 25,000 | 5,300 |
| 12. Maine | 180 | 2,900 | 6,300 |
| 13. Massachusetts | 179 | 13,900 | 29,700 |
| 14. New Hampshire | 179 | 2,300 | 4,800 |
| 15. Pennsylvania | 179 | 30,500 | 65,000 |

| | | | |
|---|---|---|---|
| 16. Indiana | 177 | 12,000 | 25,700 |
| 17. New York | 177 | 39,500 | 85,000 |
| 18. Vermont | 177 | 1,100 | 2,400 |
| 19. Alabama | 176 | 9,200 | 19,600 |
| 20. Illinois | 176 | 24,400 | 52,000 |
| 21. Michigan | 176 | 18,600 | 40,000 |
| 22. West Virginia | 176 | 4,700 | 10,000 |
| 23. Georgia | 174 | 11,900 | 25,600 |
| 24. Connecticut | 173 | 7,400 | 15,800 |
| 25. Tennessee | 173 | 10,800 | 23,200 |
| 26. Missouri | 171 | 11,600 | 24,700 |
| 27. South Carolina | 170 | 6,600 | 14,200 |
| 28. California | 168 | 52,000 | 110,000 |
| 29. Mississippi | 168 | 5,500 | 11,800 |
| 30. Arkansas | 167 | 5,700 | 12,200 |
| 31. Oregon | 167 | 6,100 | 13,000 |
| 32. North Carolina | 166 | 13,000 | 28,700 |
| 33. Oklahoma | 165 | 6,900 | 14,700 |
| 34. Washington | 165 | 8,900 | 19,100 |
| 35. Florida | 162 | 34,000 | 73,000 |
| 36. Wisconsin | 161 | 9,900 | 21,200 |
| 37. Montana | 160 | 1,600 | 3,400 |
| 38. Iowa | 158 | 6,200 | 13,000 |
| 39. Texas | 158 | 27,500 | 59,000 |
| 40. Arizona | 154 | 7,000 | 15,200 |
| 41. Minnesota | 154 | 8,300 | 17,700 |
| 42. Nebraska | 154 | 3,200 | 6,900 |
| 43. South Dakota | 153 | 1,500 | 3,200 |
| 44. Kansas | 152 | 4,900 | 10,400 |
| 45. North Dakota | 151 | 1,300 | 2,900 |
| 46. Wyoming | 149 | 700 | 1,500 |
| 47. Idaho | 146 | 1,700 | 3,600 |
| 48. Colorado | 144 | 4,800 | 10,300 |
| 49. New Mexico | 144 | 2,400 | 5,100 |
| 50. Hawaii | 138 | 1,600 | 3,500 |
| 51. Utah | 122 | 1,800 | 3,900 |

SOURCE: Data provided by the United States National Center for Health Statistics and the United States Bureau of the Census. (Figures do not reflect whether or not the age distribution is even. For example, Florida has a high cancer death rate; however, it also has a high number of seniors who have relocated there from other states.)

The usual latency period for cancer is two to forty years. The length of time during which cancer develops often makes the cause difficult or impossible to pinpoint. Where there is a specific carcinogenic agent, the lower the level of exposure, the longer the latency. For example, vinyl chloride wasn't known as a carcinogen until 1974, when an observant staff physician at B.F. Goodrich recognized a pattern of cancer in workers who had been exposed to this chemical in the 1950s. Specific causation is further complicated by the fact that cancer researchers do not yet understand why, among people who are exposed to the same carcinogens, some will get cancer and others will not.

We know that cancer can be caused by certain man-made and naturally occuring chemicals that exist in our air, water, food, homes, and in our places of work; cancer can be caused by x-rays, ultraviolet light, certain viruses, and tobacco use. Obesity, a negative response to stress, and the genes you were born with can all contribute to the development of cancer.

Fortunately, you have the power to control many of the environmental and behavioral factors that make up your lifestyle. Informed choices to change your behavior in simple, specific ways can lead to dramatically reduced cancer risks. For instance, you can choose to avoid tobacco and dietary fat, reduce repeated exposure to the sun and to cancer-causing chemicals, and learn about and begin to use techniques for reducing stress in your life. You can join activist groups that affect corporate decisions, societal actions, and government regulations. You can pressure government agencies to pass and enforce comprehensive laws that protect people from exposure to cancer-causing substances.

A number of United States government agencies have jurisdiction over the issues that relate to your health and well-being. The Occupational Safety and Health Administration (OSHA), which enforces standards of health and safety in the workplace, establishes employees' rights and employers' responsibilities, maintains records of job-related illnesses and injuries, and conducts research. The Environmental Protection Agency (EPA) administers the Toxic Substances Control Act and regulates pesticides, toxic wastes, and the contamination of air and water. The Food and Drug Administration (FDA), a branch of the United States Department of Health and Human Services, regulates food, drugs, and cosmetics. The United States Department of Agriculture (USDA) regulates certain foods such as meats and grains. The Consumer Product Safety Commission (CPSC) regulates hazards that are related to consumer products.

Your strongest allies in reducing cancer risks are a handful of private, nonprofit, action-oriented consumer-protection organizations. These include Center for Science in the Public Interest (CSPI), Citizen Action, Citizens Clearinghouse for Hazardous Wastes, Clean Water Action, Common Cause, Community Nutrition Institute, Consumers United for Food Safety, Environmental Defense Fund, Food and Water, Inc., Greenpeace, Natural Resources Defense Council (NRDC), Public Citizen Health Research Group, U.S. Public Interest Research Group (U.S.PIRG), Radioactive Waste Campaign, Sea Shepherd, and the Sierra Club.

Many of these organizations have written legislation such as the Clean Water Act and the Clean Air Act. They have funded research and pressed government agencies to enforce and strengthen existing laws. They have produced compelling reports that refute government and industry contentions that products, processes, and services that are currently on the market are harmless, and/or that the benefits of using them outweigh the risks. All too often the benefits are increased profits for manufacturers and producers, and the risks are our lives. There is absolutely no evidence that there is a safe level of exposure to any carcinogen.

Arm yourself with information and support. Do something every day to protect yourself from the risk of cancer in your food, your home, your lifestyle, and your environment. If 80 percent of cancer is linked to lifestyle, you can reduce your cancer risk by 80 percent. Cure rates for many cancer types are better than ever before, but why fight the battle when you can choose, instead, to avoid the war?

# FOOD

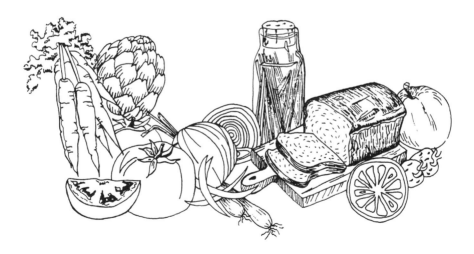

# Chapter 1

---

# ADDITIVES IN FOOD

Food additives constitute a multi-billion dollar a year business in the United States. Food additives are regulated by the federal Food and Drug Administration (FDA). The FDA also enforces the Radiation Control for Health and Safety Act (covering electronic products that emit radiation), and sections of the Public Health Service Act that relate to biological products for human use and for control of communicable diseases.

The average American diet includes at least 5,000 artificial additives each year, all of which are used for one or more of the following four purposes:

1. *To maintain or improve nutritional value,* such as through the addition of vitamins and minerals.

2. *To maintain freshness,* usually by adding sodium proprionate, potassium sorbate, and/or the antioxidants BHA (butylated hydroxyanisole) and BHT (butylated hydroxytoluene).

3. *To make food more appealing to sight* through the addition of stabilizers or artificial colors, *and to taste* through the addition of artificial flavors, sweeteners, MSG (monosodium glutamate), or other additives.

4. *To help in the processing or preparation of food* by acting in one of the following seven ways:

- as emulsifiers (mono- and diglycerides).
- as stabilizers and thickeners (gelatins and pectins).
- as pH control agents (acids and alkalizers).
- as leavening agents (baking soda).
- as maturing and bleaching agents (oxides of nitrogen, chlorine, chlorine dioxide, nitrosyl chloride).
- as anticaking agents (calcium silicate, iron ammonium citrate, silicon dioxide).
- as humectants (glycerine, sorbitol).

Some additives are safe, and some might even be beneficial. However, the government has few rules for synthetic food additives. Human testing is not required, and biochemical or behavioral effects are not considered. Over-the-counter drugs, on the other hand, are thoroughly and exhaustively studied in both human and animal tests; they must be proven to work as claimed and must not produce any harmful side effects.

Additives are regulated by the FDA under the Food, Drug and Cosmetic Act, which includes the Delaney Clause. The Delaney Clause states "that no additive shall be deemed to be safe if it is found to induce cancer when ingested by man or animal, or if it is found, after tests, which are appropriate to the evaluation of the safety of food additives, to induce cancer in man or animal . . ." Despite the clear language, under its "de minimis" policy, the FDA approves additives that cause a "relatively small" number of cancers if it is decided that the benefit of the additive outweighs the risk.

Additives are tested on animals. Large doses of a chemical are given to compensate for the small number and for the short life spans of the animals (usually rodents) that are tested. The National Cancer Institute, in its publication *Everything Doesn't Cause Cancer*, notes that:

1. Almost all proven human carcinogens cause cancer in animal tests.

2. Materials causing cancer in one species usually cause cancer in others.

3. Several known human carcinogens were first found to be carcinogenic in animals.

Public-interest groups such as Center for Science in the Public Interest (CSPI) urge stricter federal food policies, which include the following:

- The testing of the 415 chemicals that are grandfathered under the classification GRAS (Generally Regarded As Safe). This classification is based solely on the fact that these chemicals have been in use for many years.
- Granting the temporary approval of chemicals after successful animal studies, while effects on humans are evaluated.
- A limited period of licensing for approved chemicals, subject to periodic review.
- Testing of additives with other chemicals with which they will commonly be used.
- Limited, fixed terms for FDA commissioners.

The question of how chemicals interact is a critical one. In a study at California's Institute for Nutritional Studies, Dr. Benjamin Ershoff fed rats three widely used additives: sodium cyclamate, FD&C Red Dye No. 2, and polyoxyethelene sorbitran monostearate. When one chemical at a time was introduced, no changes were reported. When sodium cyclamate was fed to the rats along with Red Dye No. 2, stunted growth, hair loss, and diarrhea were observed. When all three chemicals were given, the rats lost weight rapidly and died within two weeks. (Subsequently, sodium cyclamate and FD&C Red Dye No. 2 were removed from the market because they were linked to cancer.)

Laboratory testing of an individual chemical does not reveal how the chemical may interact with other chemicals. Each chemical we ingest in our food could potentially react adversely to other chemicals in our food, as well as to chemicals to which we are exposed in the environment, in household products, and in drugs and cosmetics.

According to *The Complete Eater's Digest and Nutrition Score-board*, by Michael F. Jacobson, Ph.D., Director of CSPI, Table 1.1 presents food additives that have been linked to cancer or that are being studied as either known or suspected cancer initiators or promoters, or as causes of mutations or birth defects. Other additives listed have not yet been sufficiently studied to determine their safety so they should be avoided.

Table 1.1   Common Food Additives

| Additive | Purpose | Products |
|---|---|---|
| Acesulfame-K | Sugar substitute. | Artificially sweetened liquids, baked goods, candies. |
| Acetone peroxide | Maturing and oxidizing agent. | Baked goods. |
| Aluminum compounds, including a-ammonium sulfate; a-potassium sulfate; a-sodium sulfate; a-sulfate; sodium a-phosphate; other aluminum salts | Emulsifiers; leavening agents; neutralizing, clarifying, and firming agents. | Baked goods. |
| Arabinogalactan (larch gum) | Emulsifier; thickening agent. | Dry mixes (soups, gravies, sauces). |
| Artificial flavorings (often combinations of many chemicals) | Taste appeal. | Varied foods and beverages. |
| Artificial food colorings: Blues 1 and 2; Green 3; Reds 3 and 40; Yellows 5 and 6; Citrus Red 2 | Eye appeal. | Varied foods, especially candy, beverages, breakfast cereals, dessert powders, baked goods, ice cream, pistachio nuts, cherries, pet food, and mouthwash. (Citrus Red 2 is added only to orange skins.) |

| Additive | Purpose | Products |
|---|---|---|
| Aspartame | Sugar substitute. | Artificially sweetened foods, beverages, candy, gum (not used in cooked or baked foods). |
| Brominated vegetable oil (BVO) | Emulsifier. | Fruit-flavored soft drinks. |
| Butylated hydroxyanisole (BHA) | Antioxidant. | Varied foods, especially snack foods, cereals, chewing gum, pork sausage, lard, vegetable oils, baked goods, dry mixes. |
| Butylated hydroxytoluene (BHT) | Antioxidant. | Varied foods, especially snack foods, candy, vegetable oils and shortenings, enriched rice, and potato flakes and chips. Found in some packaging, where it migrates as a vapor into the food. |
| Caffeine | Stimulant, flavoring agent. | Coffee, cocoa, cola drinks, tea. |
| Carrageenan | Stabilizer, emulsifier. | Dairy-based products, soft drinks, ice cream, jelly, syrups, beer, sour cream, frozen whipped toppings, gelatin-type desserts, milk puddings. |
| Dioctyl sodium sulfosuccinate (DSS) | Wetting, dispersing, and solubilizing agent. | Powdered drink mixes, canned-milk beverages. |
| Hydroxylated lecithin | Emulsifier, antioxidant. | Varied foods, including baked goods, ice cream, margarine. |
| Methylene chloride | Solvent. | Some decaffeinated coffees. |
| Propyl gallate | Antioxidant. | Animal fats, vegetable oils, meat products, potato sticks, chicken-soup base, chewing gum. Sometimes added to packaging material where it migrates as a vapor into the food. |

| Additive | Purpose | Products |
|----------|---------|----------|
| Quinine | Flavoring agent. | Quinine water, bitter lemon, tonic water, and similar drinks. |
| Saccharin | Sugar substitute. | Artificially sweetened foods, gum, candy, preserves, and beverages. |
| Smoke flavoring | Flavoring agent. | Some fish, meat, nuts, and cheese. |
| Sodium nitrate, sodium nitrite | Color fixative; flavoring and antibacterial agent | Bacon, bologna, hot dogs, ham, salami, and other cured meats and fish. |
| Tannin, tannic acid | Clarifying and refining agent; flavoring agent. | Tea, coffee, cocoa, baked goods, alcoholic beverages, frozen dairy desserts, and candies; also used as an ingredient in butter, caramel, fruit, nut, brandy, and maple artificial flavorings. |
| Tertiary butylhydroquinone (TBHQ) | Antioxidant. | Varied processed foods that contain oil. |
| Xylitolsome | Sugar substitute. | Dietetic and artificially sweetened foods, gum, candy, and beverages. |

## WHAT YOU CAN DO ON A PERSONAL LEVEL

Protect yourself from harmful food additives. The following simple dietary suggestions will make a healthy difference in your life.

☐ Buy foods without added chemicals. Our contemporary lifestyles and foodstyles subject us to an inordinate number of chemicals; approximately ten thousand are available as food additives alone. Many chemicals remain in the liver for prolonged periods and can interact adversely with other ingested chemicals. This increases their harmful effects.

☐ Eat foods that are close to their natural state, ones that are locally grown and freshly picked. Choose foods that are organically grown, fed, and harvested. Foods that are unadulterated by pesticides and other petrochemicals, synthetic nutrients, or hormones of any sort are the best choices.

☐ A copy of *Eating Clean*, which deals with overcoming food hazards, including the additive avalanche, can be purchased by sending $8.00 (check or money order) to:

> *Eating Clean*
> Center for the Study of Responsive Law
> Box 19367
> Washington, DC 20036

☐ For further information on safe and unsafe food additives, and guidelines on chemical-free foods, read:

> *A Consumer Dictionary of Food Additives* by Ruth Winter. New York: Crown Publishers, 1989.

> *Poisons in Your Food* by Ruth Winter. New York: Crown Publishers, 1990.

> *Safe Food: Eating Wisely in a Risky World* by Michael Jacobson, Lisa Lefferts, and Ann Witte Garland. Los Angeles, CA: Living Planet Press, 1991.

> *Shoppers Guide to Natural Foods: A Consumers Guide to Buying and Preparing Foods for Good Health* by the editors of *East West Journal*. Garden City Park, NY: Avery Publishing Group, 1987.

## HOW TO GET MORE INVOLVED

Speak out on food issues by getting involved on a broader scale.

☐ Write a letter to the FDA urging increased and stricter controls concerning the testing and approval standards of food additives.

> Consumer Affairs
> Food and Drug Administration
> 5600 Fishers Lane – HFE 88
> Rockville, MD 20857

☐ There are many consumer-advocacy groups that urge stricter federal food policies. The following are major national organizations that lobby, pressure the FDA, and keep the public informed of the latest findings concerning food hazards.

Your questions and concerns, as well as support (either financially, or through volunteering your time and expertise), are welcomed by these groups, which are dedicated to your best interest. (Additional information on the organizations is found beginning on page 269.)

Center for Science in the
  Public Interest
Suite 300
1875 Connecticut Avenue, NW
Washington, DC 20009-5728
(202) 332-9110

Community Nutrition
  Institute
Suite 500
2001 S Street, NW
Washington, DC 20009
(202) 462-4700

Public Citizen
2000 P Street, NW
Washington, DC 20036
(202) 833-3000

# Chapter 2

# AFLATOXIN

Poisons produced by molds are known as *mycotoxins*. The most studied mycotoxin is *aflatoxin*. This potent carcinogen was first identified in 1960 when an epidemic in the British Isles killed over 100,000 farm-bred birds and animals. The source of this epidemic was finally identified as peanut meal that had been imported from Brazil. The meal had been contaminated by the common mold *Aspergillus flavus,* which produces aflatoxin.

In studies, aflatoxin has caused liver cancer in every animal species tested, including monkeys and rats. It has also caused kidney and colon cancer. The International Agency for Cancer Research (IACR) classifies aflatoxin as one of the fifty known human carcinogens. Dr. Richard Wilson, Mallinckrodt Professor of Physics at Harvard University, has referred to this mold-produced poison as "the nastiest carcinogen known to man."

Aflatoxin grows on nuts and grains, especially ones that have been weakened by drought, insects, or improper storage. Aflatoxin grows best in hot climates on crops with a high moisture content. Figure 2.1 shows how aflatoxin invades the corn plant. In developing countries where the mold is prevalent, liver-cancer rates are especially high. According to the *South African Medical Journal*, the liver-cancer rate in the Inhambane district of Mozambique is the highest in the world, as is the aflatoxin level in Inhambane's food supply.

Once the aflatoxin mold occurs, it cannot be removed; it is 100 times more potent a carcinogen than polychlorinated biphenyls

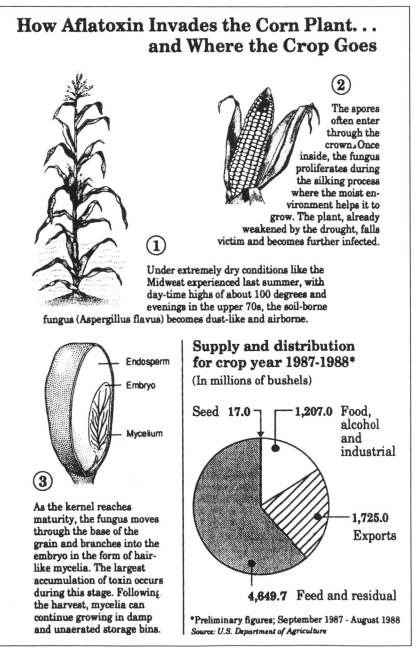

# How Aflatoxin Invades the Corn Plant...
## and Where the Crop Goes

② The spores often enter through the crown. Once inside, the fungus proliferates during the silking process where the moist environment helps it to grow. The plant, already weakened by the drought, falls victim and becomes further infected.

① Under extremely dry conditions like the Midwest experienced last summer, with day-time highs of about 100 degrees and evenings in the upper 70s, the soil-borne fungus (Aspergillus flavus) becomes dust-like and airborne.

Endosperm

Embryo

Mycelium

③ As the kernel reaches maturity, the fungus moves through the base of the grain and branches into the embryo in the form of hair-like mycelia. The largest accumulation of toxin occurs during this stage. Following the harvest, mycelia can continue growing in damp and unaerated storage bins.

## Supply and distribution for crop year 1987-1988*
(In millions of bushels)

Seed  17.0

1,207.0  Food, alcohol and industrial

1,725.0 Exports

4,649.7  Feed and residual

*Preliminary figures; September 1987 - August 1988
*Source: U.S. Department of Agriculture*

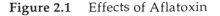

**Figure 2.1**    Effects of Aflatoxin

(PCBs). The United States Food and Drug Adminstration (FDA) has acknowledged in court depositions that there is *no safe level* of aflatoxin in foods, but the farm lobby has pressured the FDA not to impose aflatoxin controls.

The United States Department of Agriculture (USDA) inspects some corn and peanuts when they are brought to market. Samples with visible aflatoxin contamination are destroyed, as well as those that test higher than the FDA's allowable 20 ppb (parts per billion) action level. (Milk allowance is 0.5 ppb.) In years when an extremely large amount of corn exceeds the action level (enough that the FDA considers it a hardship for farming), levels of up to 100 ppb in corn animal feed and 300 ppb in cottonseed animal feed are permitted. The FDA tests a total of about 1,500 food samples each year, including 1,000 samples from lots intended for domestic use and 500 from lots intended for export by sea transport. In their book *Empty Harvest,* Dr. Bernard Jensen and Mark Anderson report that aflatoxin infestation is a direct result of using petro-type nitrogen fertilizer (anhydrous ammonia and aqueous ammonia) without replenishing the soil.

There were limited outbreaks of aflatoxin in corn in 1980 and 1983, and widespread infestations in 1977 and 1988. After a severe drought in the summer of 1988, corn crops harvested in nine major corn-producing states were found to be widely contaminated with unacceptably high levels of aflatoxin.

To reduce these high levels, the infested corn was diluted with uncontaminated corn from the 1987 harvest and it was then fed to farm animals. This resulted in hundreds of thousands of pounds of aflatoxin-contaminated milk, which had to be destroyed. In addition, Japan and the Soviet Union rejected 1988 United States corn products, while the governments of India and Guatemala lodged formal complaints over high aflatoxin levels in corn imported from the United States. To protest the 1988 United States export of contaminated corn to Mexico, in 1989 the Mexican government imported corn (and wheat and beans) from Argentina. (The USDA does not perform tests for aflatoxins on any corn that is transported by land, which is the traditional route by which the United States exports corn to Mexico.)

People consume aflatoxins primarily in corn and peanut products, and in milk from cows that eat contaminated feed. Sweet corn, the kind that we eat fresh, canned, or frozen, generally resists aflatoxin mold. Peanut, corn, and cottonseed oils are free of aflatoxin, because in the alkaline processing treatment, the mold is left behind in the grain. Due to carefully guarded growing conditions, some peanuts, such as Valencia peanuts, do not develop aflatoxins.

Foods that might contain aflatoxins are nuts, nut butters, and grains, especially corn grits, corn flour, corn meal, and corn bran. Some natural food manufacturers, such as Arrowhead Mills and Walnut Acres, submit their products regularly to the FDA, to the state, and to independent labs for testing. Aflatoxin levels in their corn and peanut products are never above 1 ppb, which is as low as the lab equipment can test. (This is certainly different from the FDA's action level of 20 ppb.)

## WHAT YOU CAN DO ON A PERSONAL LEVEL

Guard against the ingestion of aflatoxin-contaminated products. The following suggestions are offered for your protection.

☐ Before eating nuts, inspect them carefully. If they appear shriveled, moldy, discolored, or rotten, throw them away. If they taste bad, spit them out and discard the rest.

☐ Throw out any moldy grain.

☐ Consider buying products from natural food producers, such as Arrowhead Mills and Walnut Acres. Upon request, Arrowhead Mills and Walnut Acres will send you their latest product test reports and certification. They can be contacted at:

Arrowhead Mills
PO Box 2059
Hereford, TX 79045
(806) 364-0730

Walnut Acres
Walnut Acres Road
Penns Creek, PA 17862
(717) 837-0601

If you use other brands, write to the manufacturer for a copy of their latest FDA Aflatoxin Analysis Report.

## HOW TO GET MORE INVOLVED

Worried about aflatoxin levels in food and milk? Have your concerns be heard by following the suggestions provided.

☐ Express your concerns in writing to the FDA and the USDA. Urge more stringent inspection procedures and stricter controls on acceptable aflatoxin action levels.

Consumer Affairs
Food and Drug Administration
5600 Fishers Lane – HFE 88
Rockville, MD 20857

Federal Grain Inspector
U.S. Department of
  Agriculture
14th and Independence
Washington, DC 20250

☐ Find out if your state health department has developed a regular aflatoxin-inspection program for milk. If they have not, pressure your legislators. Your tax dollars pay their salaries, and their job is to represent you and your concerns.

☐ The following national organizations are active in food-safety issues, and they welcome your questions, comments, and support. Community Nutrition Institute is currently exerting pressure on the FDA to improve existing aflatoxin testing procedures and to lower aflatoxin action levels. (Additional information on the organizations is found beginning on page 269.)

Center for Science in the
  Public Interest
Suite 300
1875 Connecticut Avenue, NW
Washington, DC 20009-5728
(202) 332-9110

Community Nutrition
  Institute
Suite 500
2001 S Street, NW
Washington, DC 20009
(202) 462-4700

Public Citizen
2000 P Street, NW
Washington, DC 20036
(202) 833-3000

# Chapter 3

# ALCOHOL

Alcohol is considered to be the most dangerous legal drug known to mankind. It can damage the brain, the central nervous system, the gastrointestinal tract, the circulatory system, the musculo-skeletal system, the reproductive system, the immune system, and virtually every organ in the body. Alcohol has been linked to a long list of serious illnesses, including cancer, cirrhosis of the liver, brain damage, peptic ulcers, pneumonia, heart and coronary artery disease, vitamin deficiencies, fetal alcohol syndrome, gastritis, high blood pressure, and infection. Drinking alcohol makes osteoporosis worse; it causes metabolic damage to every cell, and it depresses immune system function. Alcohol is responsible for 60 percent of all automobile fatalities and for 10 percent of all deaths each year. Almost 33 percent of people in the United States are regular drinkers of alcoholic beverages.

According to the International Agency for Research on Cancer (IARC) of the World Health Organization, drinking alcohol has been linked to cancer of the throat, mouth, larynx, pharynx, esophagus, bladder, breast, and liver. The cancer risk is especially high for drinkers who also smoke. The *Archives of General Psychology* reported in 1990 that natural killer (NK) cell activity is reduced in people who are alcoholics as well as in people who are depressed. A dual diagnosis of alcoholism and depression lowers NK cell activity even further.

Many alcoholic beverages contain the carcinogen urethane. This cancer-causing chemical is not added intentionally to alcoholic drinks but can be formed as the result of a chemical reaction that occurs during fermentation, baking (of dessert wines), or storage.

In tests conducted by United States government agencies and the alcoholic beverage industry, high urethane levels have been found in American bourbon whiskeys; European fruit brandies; cream sherries; and in port, sake, and Chinese wine. Gin, vodka, and most domestic beers were found to have little or no urethane.

Alcoholic beverages may also contain residues of pesticides that are used to treat grapes and grains. Additionally, many wines sold in the United States contain levels of lead far higher than those allowed in drinking water. In 1991, wines tested both in the bottle and after having been poured over the lip of the bottle (where lead deposits might accumulate from the foil caps that cover the cork) produced disturbing results. When tested in the bottle, domestic wines had far lower levels of lead than imported wines, and the average lead content fell below the Environmental Protection Agency (EPA) current drinking water standard of 50 ppb (parts per billion). When the same wine was poured over the lip of the bottle, both imported and domestic wines exceeded the EPA standard. Consequently, most California wineries abandoned the practice of capping bottles with lead-foil caps after January 1, 1992.

One possible explanation for the high lead levels found in imported wines is the use of lead-soldered pipes in wine production. Another explanation is the exposure of grapes to auto exhaust in European countries, where the use of leaded gasoline and lead-contaminated groundwater are common.

Sulfites occur naturally in and are also added to wines. Sulfites inhibit spoilage during storage, and they also help prevent the wine from turning to vinegar. Many people, especially asthmatics, are allergic to sulfites. All wines bottled after 1987 must state on the labels that sulfites are present if the product contains more than 10 parts per million.

## WHAT YOU CAN DO ON A PERSONAL LEVEL

If you drink alcoholic beverages, even occasionally, consider the following suggestions.

□ Reduce your consumption of alcoholic beverages. The United States Department of Health and Human Services recommends that you drink two or fewer alcoholic drinks each day, but many physicians believe this recommendation is too high. (A drink is considered to be one 12-ounce can of beer, one 5-ounce glass of wine, or 1½ ounces of spirits.)

□ Drink organic wines that are not contaminated by pesticides. A number of large California wineries, including Gallo, Fetzer, Sutter Home, and Buena Vista, as well as some smaller wineries, including Four Chimneys Farm, Frey Brothers, and the Organic Wine Works of Santa Cruz, are converting a large portion of their acreage to organic crops. Wine makers do not usually label their wine "organic," however, because of the concern that an organic label might generate confusion among consumers, or could imply that non-organic wines are not safe. Information on organic wines is available from

Organic Grapes into Wine Alliance
54 Genoa Place
San Francisco, CA 94133
(800) 477-0167
(415) 433-0167

□ When you open a bottle of wine, before pouring it, remove the foil cap and wipe the lip of the bottle with a cloth or paper towel that has been moistened with water, vinegar, or lemon juice. This will remove traces of lead that have been left by the cap. Make sure this is done before the wine is poured. Be aware that bottles with leaky corks may have already allowed the wine to come into contact with and react to the lead-foil caps.

□ Never store alcoholic beverages in lead-crystal decanters and never drink alcohol from lead-crystal glasses. Tests have shown that lead levels more than doubled in one hour—increasing from

33 ppb to 68 ppb—in white wine that had been sitting in a lead-crystal goblet. The lead level of port wine stored in a crystal decanter for four months increased from 89 ppb to over 2,162 ppb.

☐  If you have or know someone who has a drinking problem, contact an alcoholism treatment center for help. These centers are listed in most local yellow pages under *Alcoholism Information and Treatment Centers.*

☐  For more information, including the urethane test results of many brands of alcoholic beverages, read: *Tainted Booze: The Consumer's Guide to Urethane in Alcoholic Beverages* by Charles Mitchell and Michael Jacobson. This book can be found in most local libraries or can be purchased by sending a check or money order in the amount of $3.95 (price includes shipping and handling) along with your request to:

Center for Science in the Public Interest
Publication Department
Suite 300
1875 Connecticut Avenue, NW
Washington, DC 20009-5728

## HOW TO GET MORE INVOLVED

Become aware and actively involved with issues concerning alcoholic beverages. Let your voice be heard.

☐  Contact your local school administrators and PTA members. Urge them to include alcohol- and drug-awareness programs as part of their regular curriculum. Many police precincts across the country sponsor free in-school programs such as DARE (Drug Abuse Resistance Education) and PRIDE (Peer Resistance Instruction Drug Education). These seminars help make children aware of the dangers of drugs and alcohol. In addition, they help children resist peer pressure.

☐  Write letters to local, state, and federal legislators urging them to pass laws requiring the ingredients and caloric content of alcoholic beverages to be indicated on labels. Demand explicit health-risk warnings on labels. Warnings should include increased risk of cancer and other serious diseases.

☐ Support consumer-protection groups that work to establish protective alcohol policies. The following national organizations are involved with issues such as drunk driving, underage drinking, and the raising of sales tax on alcoholic beverages (making them less affordable for young people). These groups also encourage a change in the advertising of alcohol, as well as the promotion of stronger warnings on labels. (Additional information on the organizations is found beginning on page 269.)

Center for Science in the
  Public Interest
Suite 300
1875 Connecticut Avenue, NW
Washington, DC 20009-5728
(202) 332-9110

Mothers Against Drunk
  Driving (MADD)
PO Box 541688
Dallas, TX 75354-1688
(214) 744-MADD

National Council on Alcoholism and Drug Dependence
12 West 21st Street
New York, NY
(800) NCA-CALL

# Chapter 4

# CAFFEINE

Caffeine is an ingredient that is naturally present in coffee beans; tea; cacao seeds, from which cocoa and chocolate are made; betel nuts; and cola nuts, used to produce cola beverages and some medicines. Caffeine is also added to many soft drinks, which are the major source of caffeine in the United States for both adults and children.

Caffeine has been linked to bladder cancer, pancreatic cancer, and fibrocystic breast disease (benign breast lumps). Women with fibrocystic breast disease run an increased risk of developing breast cancer. These benign cysts have also been known to camouflage malignant tumors. In some cases, fibrocystic breast disease has reversed within six months to two years once all caffeine was withdrawn from the diet.

Caffeine is also a known animal *teratogen* (the cause of birth defects). In studies, animals that have been fed large amounts of caffeine have produced offspring with cleft palates, missing fingers and toes, and skull malformations. A 1980 study sponsored by the Center for Science in the Public Interest (CSPI) indicated that women who drink eight or more cups of coffee daily may have a higher risk of bearing children with birth defects. When caffeine is combined with other chemical teratogens, it may react synergistically, heightening negative effects.

In addition to caffeine, some coffee contains pesticides as well. A 1983 study by the Natural Resources Defense Council (NRDC) found that 30 percent of green (unroasted) and roasted coffee beans contained pesticide residues when tested by standard FDA methods.

Subsequent tests using improved detection methods found that 100 percent of unroasted coffee beans were contaminated with such pesticides as DDT, lindane, aldrin, and chlordane. Although these pesticides are banned for use in the United States, many coffee-producing countries impose no regulations for these chemicals.

Decaffeinated coffee, on the other hand, contains approximately one-twentieth the amount of caffeine that is found in regular coffee, but the chemical frequently used in the decaffeination process—methylene chloride—has been linked specifically to lung and liver cancer. (While permitting methylene chloride in coffee, the FDA has banned it in hairsprays, an inscrutable decision since more people drink coffee than use hairspray.)

If you drink tea in large amounts, unless it is herbal tea, you might also be at risk from the ingestion of too much *tannin* (tannic acid), a suspected human carcinogen. Tannin occurs naturally in a variety of plants, including tea leaves; it is also present in insignificant amounts in coffee and cocoa. Tannin has been linked to oral and esophageal cancer in the populations of many countries. However, a number of studies, including several that were done at the Chinese Academy of Preventive Medicine in Beijing, have also shown that green tea, consumed mostly in Japan and China, is rich in unoxidized *polyphenols*. Polyphenols inhibit the action of many cancer-causing chemicals. This may account for the fact that Japanese people who are heavy green-tea drinkers have lower death rates from all types of cancer, including stomach cancer—a major killer in Japan.

Americans consume an average of over thirty gallons of soft drinks a year. Because of differences in body weight, a 12-ounce caffeinated soda has the same effect on a child that a 6-ounce cup of coffee has on an adult. A child who drinks several caffeinated sodas a day might become jittery and experience insomnia. In addition to caffeine, most sodas contain large amounts of sugar and/or artificial sweeteners.

## WHAT YOU CAN DO ON A PERSONAL LEVEL

Reduce health risks resulting from caffeine by making some simple changes.

☐ Do not drink more than one cup of a caffeinated beverage a day. Pregnant women should avoid caffeine entirely.

☐ Look for organic (pesticide-free) coffee in natural foods stores. Organic coffee can also be purchased through mail-order companies, such as:

Clean Foods, Inc.
PO Box 1647
Ojai, CA 93024
(800) 526-8328
(805) 646-5535

Walnut Acres
Walnut Acres Road
Penns Creek, PA, 17862
(717) 837-0601

Royal Blue Organics Cafe Organico is grown by the farmers of a cooperative of peasants of Mayan descent. This coffee is certified "organic" by the Biodynamic Association of Brazil. Twenty percent of profits from the sales of Cafe Organico go to the Northwest Coalition for Alternatives to Pesticides (NCAP).

Royal Blue Organics
28718 Royal Avenue
Eugene, OR 97402
(503) 689-1836

☐ If you drink decaffeinated coffee, read the label. Make sure the coffee has been water-decaffeinated. High Point, Taster's Choice, and Nescafé are good choices.

☐ Add milk to your tea. Milk binds tannin, so it cannot be absorbed by the body.

☐ Switch to caffeine-free sodas. The best brands are those without artificial flavors, colors, or sweeteners.

☐ Drink herbal teas, but not teas that contain comfrey, coltsfoot, or sassafras. These herbs have been linked to cancer. Because of this concern, sassafras was banned from food in 1960.

## HOW TO GET MORE INVOLVED

Awareness of the possible health hazards of caffeinated foods and beverages is your best weapon. There is, however, something else you can do on a broader scale.

☐ Support organizations that focus attention either on nutritional awareness of foods and beverages, or on the reduction of dangerous pesticide use on crops. (Additional information on the organizations is found beginning on page 269.)

Center for Science in the
  Public Interest
Suite 300
1875 Connecticut Avenue, NW
Washington, DC 20009-5728
(202) 332-9110

Community Nutrition
  Institute
Suite 500
2001 S Street, NW
Washington, DC 20009
(202) 462-4700

National Coalition Against the
  Misuse of Pesticides
Suite 200
701 E Street, SE
Washington, DC 20003
(202) 543-5450

Northwest Coalition for
  Alternatives to Pesticides
PO Box 1393
Eugene, OR 97440
(503) 344-5044

# Chapter 5

# DIETARY FAT

In the typical American diet, 40 percent of calories come from fat. While the National Cancer Institute (NCI) has recommended that Americans get no more than 30 percent of their calories from fat, early results of an ongoing NCI-sponsored study of diet in China suggest that only 10 to 15 percent of calories should come from fat. This study, begun in 1983, is considered the most comprehensive diet study ever undertaken (the New York Times columnist Jane E. Brody referred to it as "the Grand Prix of epidemiology"). It is just as important to note that if less than 10 percent of calories come from fat, there is the risk of essential fatty acid deficiency.

In a 1990 study reported by the American Health Foundation, it was concluded that a high-fat, low-fiber diet increased cancer risk, especially cancer of the colon. *The Journal of the National Cancer Institute* reported in 1990 that a high-fat diet that is also low in carbohydrates, fiber, and vitamin C correlates with a positive prognosis for breast cancer. High-fat diets have also been proven to suppress immune-system responses in laboratory animals. An American Health Foundation study found that a lean diet promotes production of the immune system's natural killer cells. Men who reduced their fat intake by 9 percent (from 32 percent to 23 percent) showed a 49 percent increase in immune-cell activity.

High temperatures that are used in commercial processing and in cooking—including the cooking of many prepared and packaged foods—can damage fats by converting polyunsaturates from the beneficial *cis* form of fat to *trans* fats, which can create weakened, permeable cell membranes that disarm the body's immune system. We need a healthy immune system to help kill cancer cells, which are present from time to time in each of our bodies.

Fats can also be damaged by *hydrogenation* and *oxidation*. Hydrogenation converts liquid oils to solid forms of fat such as margarine. Hydrogenated fats contain fatty-acid fragments and altered molecules that are created from fatty acids. These fragments and molecules could be toxic. Fats can also be contaminated by the metal catalyst (nickel, copper, or platinum) that is used in the hydrogenation process. Total hydrogenation of fats creates substances that do not spoil, that can be given any desired texture, and that have no essential-fatty-acid activity (they will not convert from the cis form of fat to a trans fat). Partial hydrogenation of fats produces a spectrum of chemicals that vary in content and number from batch to batch. It is impossible to control the production of these compounds during the partial-hydrogenation process, but these compounds include trans-fatty acids that can lower immune-system function. Most of these compounds have not been studied for their effects on health. Many consumer food advocates believe that if the process of partial hydrogenation—which has been in use since the 1930s—was introduced today, the Food and Drug Administration would not approve it.

Oxidation takes place when fats or oils are manufactured or stored improperly. Most oxidized fats and oils taste rancid. Oxidation leads to the formation of *free radicals*. These highly active molecules can attack and disrupt the vital chain of oxygen and can alter the body's DNA and RNA (nucleic acids that are responsible for genetic traits). These mutations could result in cancer unless antioxidants are present to check and neutralize the process. Unfortunately, the naturally occurring protective antioxidants in these oils are lost during refining.

It is important to keep dietary fat intake below 30 percent of total calories consumed (ideally between 10 and 15 percent). To determine the percentage of calories that come from fat, use the following formula:

1. Multiply the grams of fat per serving by 9 (there are 9 calories in a gram of fat), then divide the resulting number by the total calories per serving. For example, let's say one serving of a particular food has a total of 360 calories, containing 10 grams of fat. First, multiply 10 (total grams of fat) times 9 (calories per gram) to reach the number 90 (total fat calories).

$$
\begin{array}{rl}
10 & \text{total grams of fat} \\
\underline{\times\,9} & \text{calories per gram} \\
90 & \text{total calories from fat}
\end{array}
$$

2. Next, divide 90 (total calories from fat) by 360 (total serving calories) to arrive at .25 or 25 percent. In this example, 25 percent of calories come from fat.

$$
\begin{array}{rl}
90 & \text{total calories from fat} \\
\underline{\div\,360} & \text{total serving calories} \\
.25 & \text{total calories in this serving} \\
 & \text{that come from fat}
\end{array}
$$

Essential fats are important to include in one's diet; they regulate the immune system, and the body cannot manufacture them. These fats are the Omega-3 fatty acid EPA (eicosapentaenoic acid) and the Omega-6 fatty acid GLA (gamma linolenic acid).

Omega-6 oils (GLA) come from evening primrose oil, black currant seeds, borage, gooseberries, and spirulina. Unrefined vegetable oils, especially safflower and sunflower oils, contain high amounts of cis-linoleic acid, which can convert to GLA in the body. GLA plays a direct role in cancer prevention. The body requires GLA in order to produce hormone-like compounds known as *prostaglandins*, including the prostaglandin known as PGE1, which helps regulate the thymus gland and the cancer-killing T-lymphocyte cells of the immune system.

Prostaglandin production also requires certain enzyme co-factors: vitamin B3 (niacin and niacinamide), vitamin B6 (pyridoxine), vitamin C, magnesium, and zinc. Prostaglandins made from GLA have been found to slow the growth rate of breast cancer and to stimulate cancer cells to revert back to normal cells.

A report in the *Journal of the National Cancer Institute* (1989) stated that Omega-3 oils (EPA) provided protection against breast, colon, and pancreatic cancer. These oils are found in many cold-water fish and seafoods, especially anchovies, salmon, herring, mackerel, tuna, and halibut. Trace amounts of EPA are found in some leafy green vegetables, such as purslane—a green that is used frequently in soups and salads in Mediterranean countries—in soybeans, and in canola oil. The EPA precursor ALA (alpha-linolenic acid) also enhances prostaglandin production, and is found in wheat sprouts, wheat germ, wheat nuts, linseeds, flaxseeds, and soybeans.

Unprocessed polyunsaturated oils (corn, cottonseed, hazelnut, safflower, sesame, soy, sunflower, and walnut)—in their unrefined and unheated states—are excellent sources of the essential fatty acid GLA. Unprocessed oils are labeled "expeller pressed," "crude," or "unrefined." These oils are extracted from the plant material that bears them in a unique process. First, the plant material is ground or flaked, and then it is placed in a large cylinder. A revolving worm shaft presses the material against the walls of the cylinder and a back plate. This pressure releases the oil, which is then expelled through slots in the cylinder.

Processed oils, on the other hand, are generally extracted from their sources by grinding the plants' seeds and bathing them in a solvent. The most commonly used solvent is hexane, which is derived from petroleum. This method is economical for producers because nearly 100 percent of the oil is extracted and very little residue remains, but ingesting a petroleum product is as unhealthy as it is unappetizing.

Mono-unsaturated oils (olive, peanut, and canola) remain stable at high heat and are, therefore, safe to cook with. Olive oils are labeled "extra virgin," "virgin," and pure." Extra virgin and virgin oils are more expensive because they are made with the most select olives and come from the first pressing. Pure olive oil is a combination of refined oils from later pressings.

## WHAT YOU CAN DO ON A PERSONAL LEVEL

The following suggestions are offered to lower health risks that may result from too much dietary fat.

☐ Reduce the amount of fat in your diet. Your fat intake should be between 10 and 15 percent of the total calories consumed. (See formula on page 35 for determining the percentage of calories that come from fat.)

☐ Include the essential fats EPA and GLA in your diet.

☐ For salads and cold dishes use unprocessed, polyunsaturated oils (corn, cottonseed, hazelnut, safflower, sesame, soy, sunflower, and walnut).

☐ When cooking, use mono-unsaturated oils (olive, peanut, and canola).

☐ If you frequently eat in restaurants, eat fast foods or commercially prepared foods at home, or if you don't eat fish, consider taking supplements that contain essential oils. Omega-3 oil supplements are sold as linseed oil, flaxseed oil, and EPA capsules. Use only linseed-oil supplements that are formulated for consumption. Never use linseed oil formulated for use on wood, because it contains toxic additives, including lead. Omega-6 oil supplements are sold as evening primrose oil and safflower oil capsules. The most beneficial effects are produced when twice as much Omega-6 as Omega-3 oil is consumed.

☐ For maximum benefits, GLA-producing foods and supplements shouldn't be taken together with ALA sources (wheat sprouts, wheat germ, wheat nuts, linseeds, flaxseed, soybeans) because ALA inhibits GLA prostaglandin production.

☐ If you include essential oils in your diet, you may enjoy the added benefit of stabilizing your optimum weight—essential oils help burn calories more efficiently—and of reducing your cholesterol level and risk of cardiovascular disease.

☐ For further information on dietary fat, read:

*Beyond Pritikin* by Ann Louise Gittleman. New York: Bantam Books, 1988.

*Cancer and Nutrition: A Ten Point Plan to Reduce Your Chances of Getting Cancer* by Charles B. Simone, M.D. Garden City Park, NY: Avery Publishing Group, 1992.

*Making Fats and Oils Work for You* by Lewis Harrison. Garden City Park, NY: Avery Publishing Group, 1990.

*The Complete & Up-to-Date Fat Book* by Karen J. Bellerson. Garden City Park, NY: Avery Publishing Group, 1990.

## HOW TO GET MORE INVOLVED

Take an active part in showing your concern on issues dealing with health and nutrition.

☐ Support organizations that keep the public informed of important nutritional breakthroughs and other health-related information. The following national organizations are actively involved in issues concerning food and nutrition. (Additional information on the organizations is found beginning on page 269.)

Center for Science in the
  Public Interest
Suite 300
1875 Connecticut Avenue, NW
Washington, DC 20009-5728
(202) 332-9110

Community Nutrition
  Institute
Suite 500
2001 S Street, NW
Washington, DC 20009
(202) 462-4700

Public Citizen
2000 P Street, NW
Washington, DC 20036
(202) 833-3000

# Chapter 6

# DIETARY IMBALANCE

According to the Department of Health and Human Services, at least one-third of all cancers may be linked to what we eat, while the National Academy of Sciences feels that up to 60 percent of cancer may be diet-related. (In 1991, the National Cancer Institute announced a five-year, $6.3 million program to research and develop foods that might protect against cancer.)

Although cancer rates vary widely among different countries, when people of one race or ethnic origin move to another country and adopt that country's diet, their risk of getting cancer follows the predictable patterns that exist in the new location. This has led researchers to conclude that although some cancers develop in response to genetic predisposition, it is more likely that environmental and dietary factors are the catalysts for the development of most cancers.

In April 1991, the Physicians Committee for Responsible Medicine proposed that the United States Department of Agriculture (USDA) replace the basic four food groups—meat, poultry, and fish; dairy and eggs; fruits and vegetables; and breads and cereals—with a diet of whole grains, vegetables, legumes, and fruits. The committee pointed out that most major diet-related diseases in the United States are extremely rare in developing countries, where little or no meat and few dairy products are eaten.

Shortly thereafter, the USDA proposed a new four-level

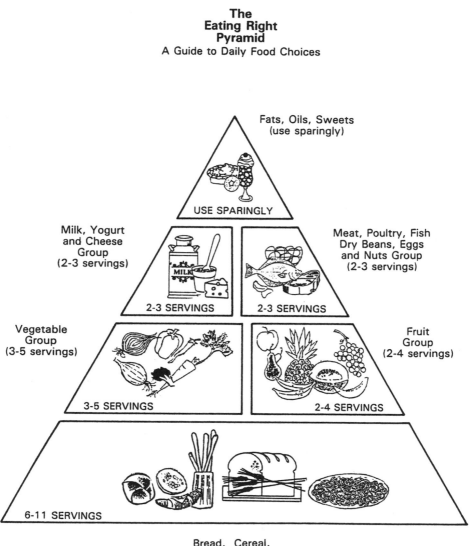

**Figure 6.1** Current USDA Food Guide Pyramid (originally proposed as the Eating Right Pyramid).

Eating Right Pyramid (see Figure 6.1), which had been developed over a three-year period and reviewed by the United States Department of Health and Human Services. Grains—including bread, cereal, and pasta—formed the broad base of the pyramid (6 to 11 servings daily). The narrower, second layer included fruits (3 to 5 servings daily) and vegetables (2 to 4 servings daily), followed by a layer of dairy products (2 to 3 servings daily) and meat, fish, poultry, eggs, legumes, and nuts (2 to 3 servings daily). The small, triangular top level included fats, oils, and sweets, which were "to be used sparingly."

Ten days after announcing the Eating Right Pyramid, the Secretary of Agriculture cancelled the program, allegedly because children might find the pyramid graphic confusing. However, according to Gerald Combs, former chairman of the USDA Subcommittee for Human Nutrition, the Eating Right Pyramid was cancelled under intense political pressure from self-interest groups.

The National Cattlemen's Association (NCA) and the National Milk Producers' Federation (NMPF) complained that the number of recommended servings of their products was smaller than the recommended servings of vegetables, fruits, and bread; and that their position on the chart near fats implied a judgment among the food groups. (NCA has taken credit for influencing the Secretary of Agriculture.)

The USDA nutritionists who developed the food-guide pyramid were not consulted about or permitted to comment on its cancellation, and the scheduled presentations of consumer research that supported the pyramid were cancelled. Nonetheless, many experts on nutrition continued to believe that the Eating Right Pyramid recommended clearly and accurately the appropriate number of servings that should be consumed from each food group.

In April 1992, one year (and $1 million) after its initial debut, the USDA officially replaced the four food groups with the Food Guide Pyramid. This graphic is now the primary device for educating the public about nutrition.

In its 1987 publication *Diet, Nutrition and Cancer Prevention: A Guide to Food Choices*, the United States Department of Health and Human Services, the Public Health Service, and the National Institutes of Health, recommend that we eat a variety of foods for proper nutritional intake and balance. No single food or family of foods contains all the nutrients we need.

### WHAT YOU CAN DO ON A PERSONAL LEVEL

Eat well-balanced, nutritious meals. The following suggestions will help you accomplish this goal.

☐ Eat just enough calories to maintain your desired weight. NIH recommends that 10–20 percent of total daily calories come from protein. Most people in the United States eat a great deal more protein than this. Another 10–20 percent should come from fat, and 60–80 percent should be from complex carbohydrates. Eat more grains, fruits, and vegetables; eat fewer animal products, fats, and sugars. Eliminate refined and processed foods because they usually contain fewer nutrients. Eat slowly and chew food thoroughly.

☐ Include the following foods in your diet, which (according to studies) contain cancer- and radiation-fighting properties: sea vegetables (arame, kombu, wakame, nori), fermented foods (miso, tempeh, shoyu, tamari), grains, beets, dried primary-grown nutritional yeast, garlic, mono-unsaturated oils (peanut, olive, canola), and foods rich in chlorophyll (sprouts, celery, leafy greens, broccoli, spirulina, parsley). Combine grains and legumes to make whole proteins. If you do not eat meat or dairy products, be sure to include good sources of zinc, calcium, and vitamin $B_{12}$ (these can be taken in supplement form) in your diet.

☐ For more information on a healthy, cancer-prevention diet, read:

*Cancer and Nutrition: A Ten Point Plan to Reduce Your Chances of Getting Cancer* by Charles B. Simone, M.D. Garden City Park, NY: Avery Publishing Group, 1992.

*Dr. Moerman's Anti-Cancer Diet* by Ruth Jochem. Garden City Park, NY: Avery Publishing Group, 1990.

*Food and Healing* by Annmarie Colbin. New York: Ballantine Books, 1986.

*Safe Food: Eating Wisely in a Risky World*, by Michael F. Jacobson, Lisa Y. Lefferts, and Anne Witte Garland. Los Angeles: Living Planet Press, 1991.

*What's in My Food: A Book of Nutrients* by Xandria Williams. Garden City Park, NY: Prism Press, 1988.

## HOW TO GET MORE INVOLVED

Show your concern regarding issues on food and nutrition by getting more involved.

☐ Support organizations that keep the public informed on important nutritional breakthroughs and other health-related information. The following national organizations are actively involved in issues concerning food and nutrition. (Additional information on the organizations is found beginning on page 269.)

Center for Science in the
 Public Interest
Suite 300
1875 Connecticut Avenue, NW
Washington, DC 20009-5728
(202) 332-9110

Community Nutrition
 Institute
Suite 500
2001 S Street, NW
Washington, DC 20009
(202) 462-4700

Public Citizen
2000 P Street, NW
Washington, DC 20036
(202) 833-3000

# Chapter 7

# IRRADIATION OF FOOD

After World War II, President Dwight D. Eisenhower initiated a program known as Atoms for Peace. This program—now known as the Department of Energy (DOE) Byproducts Utilization Program—was designed to find peaceful uses for nuclear waste. Atoms for Peace ultimately generated both the nuclear-power and nuclear-medicine industries, and led to the initial DOE funding in 1953 of studies on food irradiation.

Food irradiation uses ionizing radiation from radioactive isotopes (cesium-137 or cobalt-60) or from devices that produce beta or x-rays to treat fresh food. The irradiation process lengthens the shelf life of fresh foods by inhibiting sprouting, delaying ripening and mold growth, reducing the number of insects and microorganisms that can lead to rotting, killing certain types of bacteria, and rendering harmless a number of disease-causing parasites such as trichinae. High doses of radiation can sterilize food for hospital patients, including organ-transplant patients, for whom a microbiologically sterile diet is prescribed.

In an irradiation plant, food is placed on a conveyor belt and passed from the loading facility to the irradiation cell, where it is exposed to the radiation source. The distance of the food from the radiation source and the length of exposure time are factors that determine how great the radiation dose is. After irradiation, the food moves to a storage facility where it awaits relocation to long-term storage or to retailers.

The unit of received dose of irradiation is called a rad. Irradiation levels range from 15,000 rads to kill enzymes in sprouting potatoes to 3 million rads to kill bacteria in spices (this is 60 million times the radiation dose delivered by a standard 0.05 rad chest x-ray).

Foods do not become radioactive as a result of being irradiated. However, irradiation rearranges the molecular structure of food, and may promote the formation of toxic radiolytic products such as the carcinogens aflatoxin and formaldehyde. Some radiolytic products are formed that are unique to irradiated foods; these toxic by-products are known as URPs (unique radiolytic products). The long-term effects of ingesting URPs are simply not yet known.

Also, gamma radiation can deplete or destroy essential nutrients in foods, including vitamins A, B, C, E, and K; amino acids; fats and fatty acids; carbohydrates; enzymes; and nucleic acids (the genetic carriers that are the basis for cell division, growth, and development). The higher the radiation dose, the greater the nutrient loss or damage.

There is some concern that mutations produced by irradiation may induce the development of resistant microbiological strains. Additionally, irradiation can cause discoloration of meats, unpleasant flavor in fruits, meats, and dairy products, and a mushy consistency in produce.

Irradiation destroys microorganisms that cause rotting food to smell bad, so food that smells fresh may actually be rotten. Irradiation can cause mutations in bacteria that may lead to the creation of new strains of pest organisms. Furthermore, nuclear reactions in irradiated food induce the formation of artificial atom types, some of which are radioactive.

Clearly, a reduction in the amount of pesticides used worldwide in food agriculture is a desirable goal; but there may be preferable biotechnological alternatives to irradiation, such as the development of pesticide-resistant crops. In the meantime, there is presently no way to prove that food irradiation is safe. The FDA waived its customary requirement of animal testing, and based its approval of food irradiation on theoretical calculations from radiation chemistry and physics. The FDA stated that adequate toxicological studies could not be done, and that "studies of sufficiently high quality to support the safety of irradiated foods . . . are also not available."

The first irradiation facility built solely to irradiate food opened in Mulberry, Florida, in January 1992. Prior to the opening of the Mulberry plant, the only foods irradiated in the United States were spices (approximately 5 percent of which were treated). Most of the forty operating irradiation facilities in the United States now sterilize disposable medical products (as well as spices). The FDA plans to turn these facilities into food processing plants; it also plans to build 1,000 additional plants and mobile units (an average of twenty in each state) with the capacity to irradiate half our food supply. These radiation facilities, which will be built in urban neighborhoods as well as in rural and farming communities, will have between one million and ten million curies of radioactive material on site. (Ten million curies of cesium-137 is more than 1,000 times the cesium released by a 20-kiloton nuclear bomb.)

Cobalt-60 is hazardous for 50 to 100 years, and cesium-137 is hazardous for 300 to 600 years. In addition, cesium-137 is water-soluble. When cesium-137 leaches into groundwater supplies, it is virtually impossible to contain it or to make the water pure again. Large quantities of these and other radioactive materials required for the food irradiation process will be transported on the nation's highways and railroads from nuclear production and storage sites to irradiation plants.

The increase in volume of these radioactive shipments means a commensurate increase in the chances that there will be an even greater number of accidental spills of hazardous materials every year. (The number of spills from rail cars alone increased by 46 percent between 1985 and 1991. In 1990, there were 1,228 rail accidents and 7,214 highway accidents that resulted in hazardous waste spills; most road accidents occured due to the same causes that produce non-nuclear accidents: careless driving, driver fatigue, dangerous road conditions, excessive speed, and deer or elk on the highway at night.)

At a Center for Science in the Public Interest (CSPI) forum in October 1987, food-irradiation proponent Dr. Ari Brynjolffs accurately, if inadvertently, summed up the government's case: "Food irradiation is good for food, because it is so dangerous for everything that is living." Many independent scientists and consumers nationwide concur that, indeed, food irradiation may be very dangerous for everything that is living, including human beings; they believe government approval of food irradiation is premature.

## WHAT YOU CAN DO ON A PERSONAL LEVEL

If you are concerned with the possible harms of irradiated foods, follow the suggestions given.

☐ Don't buy irradiated whole foods, which you can identify by a radura symbol—a flower in a circle with the words "treated with radiation" (see Figure 7.1).

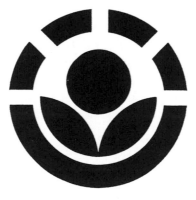

**Figure 7.1**   Radura Symbol

☐ Express your feelings concerning irradiated foods to your local grocery-store manager. Insist that if he sells irradiated foods, they be clearly labeled. Also ask that a line of non-irradiated foods be provided, as well.

☐ Unfortunately, ingredients in processed foods and ingredients used in restaurants do not have to be identified. Food and Water, Inc., which is a national organization working to prevent food irradiation, publishes a list of large food companies, supermarkets, poultry companies, and fast food restaurants that have stated that they do not and will not use radiation-exposed foods. To receive a copy of this list and to obtain additional information on food irradiation, contact:

Food and Water, Inc.
225 Lafayette Street – Suite 613
New York, NY 10012
(800) EAT-SAFE
(212) 941-9340

☐ Be aware of the FDA's list of foods that have been authorized for irradiation:

| | |
|---|---|
| Dried enzyme preparations | Seafood |
| Fruits | Vegetables |
| Pork | Wheat |
| Poultry | Wheat flour |

Dried herbs and spices:

| | | |
|---|---|---|
| Allspice | Dill weed | Parsley |
| Anise | Fennel seeds | Pepper (black |
| Basil | Fenugreek | and white) |
| Bay leaves | Garlic powder | Red pepper |
| Caraway seeds | Ginger | Peppermint |
| Black cumin | Grains of paradise | Poppy seeds |
| Cardamom | Horseradish | Rosemary |
| Celery seeds | Mace | Saffron |
| Chamomile | Marjoram | Sage |
| Chervil | Mustard seeds | Savory |
| Chives | Mustard flour | Sesame seeds |
| Cinnamon | Nutmeg | Spearmint |
| Cloves | Onion powder | Star anise seeds |
| Coriander | Orange petals | Tarragon |
| Cumin seeds | Oregano | Thyme |
| Dill seeds | Paprika | Turmeric |

## HOW TO GET MORE INVOLVED

If you are concerned with current food-irradiation policies, you have the power to take a stand and make a difference.

☐  Write to elected officials and urge them to support bills that call for:

- the halting of food irradiation until further studies are done.
- the labeling of irradiated ingredients used in processed foods.
- stricter monitoring requirements of irradiation facilities.

Your Senators
United States Senate
Washington, DC 20204

Your Representatives
House of Representatives
Washington, DC 20515

☐  A letter voicing your concerns on food irradiation is a powerful tool. Express your feelings to the following government agencies.

Department of Health
  and Human Services
Hubert H. Humphrey Bldg.
200 Independence Avenue, SW
Washington, DC 20201

Petitions Control Branch
Food and Drug Administration
200 C Street, SW
Washington, DC 20204

☐  Actively support organizations that either lobby against or work to promote stricter testing of irradiated foods by the FDA. These groups are also sources of the most current findings on food irradiation. (Additional information on the organizations is found beginning on page 269.)

Center for Science in the
  Public Interest
Suite 300
1875 Connecticut Avenue, NW
Washington, DC 20009-5728
(202) 332-9110

Food and Water
Suite 613
225 Lafayette Street
New York, NY 10012
(800) EAT-SAFE
(212) 941-9340

# Chapter 8

# LACK OF DIETARY FIBER

Dietary fiber is an important component of a balanced diet. High-fiber foods were once staples of the American diet, but in the early decades of the twentieth century they were proportionately displaced by refined sugars and fats. The importance of high-fiber foods was redicovered in the late 1960s, largely due to the research conducted in Africa by Dr. Denis Burkitt. He observed that among rural Africans who were on a high-fiber diet, cancer and heart disease were virtually unknown. In addition, Ugandans, whose diet supplied an average of 25 grams of fiber per day, never experienced the common American problems of constipation, hiatal hernias, and varicose veins. Since his work was first published, the beneficial effects of fiber have been widely reported.

Dietary fiber is nondigestible material from plants, including grains, legumes, fruits, and vegetables. Because fiber is either poorly digested or not able to be digested at all, it has no direct nutritional value; it is, nonetheless, of great benefit to your health. Fiber helps speed food and the by-products of digestion through the large intestine and out of the body. A shorter bowel transit time means that toxins are removed from the body quickly, including bile acids, which are formed by the liver to break down fats and oils for digestion in the intestine. When bile acids remain in contact with the intestinal wall for too long a period of time, they can develop into cancer-causing substances. Fiber helps provide protection against cancers of the colon, rectum, stomach, lungs, esophagus, mouth, and breast.

The typical American diet supplies approximately 15 grams of fiber each day. The National Cancer Insitute recommends increasing one's fiber intake to 30 grams daily. Consumer nutrition advocates recommend increasing fiber intake to at least 40 grams each day. In countries where a high-fiber diet is consumed, there are lower rates of cancer, particularly cancers of the colon, breast, and rectum. Results of a study published in the 1991 *Journal of the National Cancer Institute* suggest that breast-cancer rates can be significantly reduced by doubling the amount of fiber in the diet.

Another study reported in the 1991 *Journal of the National Cancer Institute* found that a diet that included 20 to 30 grams of wheat bran fiber per day specifically protected against cancers of the breast and colon. The reasons for this finding may be two-fold: according to a 1991 American Health Foundation study, a diet high in wheat bran is associated with lower levels of circulating estrogen, which can promote the growth and development of some breast cancers; similar amounts of corn bran and/or oat bran did not lower estrogen levels. Another American Health Foundation study that examined the effects of wheat, corn, and oat bran found that only wheat fiber produced significantly lowered levels of the secondary bile acids and bacterial enzymes that can promote colon cancer.

There are seven kinds of fiber: bran, cellulose, hemicellulose, lignin, pectin, gums, and mucilages. All fibers can help remove cancer-causing substances from the colon, help maintain steady blood sugar, and help prevent heart disease by reducing cholesterol, triglycerides, and low-density lipoprotein levels. In addition, pectin can help the body eliminate lead and other heavy metals. All fruits, vegetables, legumes, and whole grain foods contain varying amounts of fiber and should be included in the daily diet. Specific sources of fiber are presented in Table 8.1.

Dr. T. Colin Campbell of Cornell University, who leads the largest ongoing study of diet ever undertaken, states, "We're basically a vegetarian species, and [we] should be eating a wide variety of plant foods and minimizing our intake of animal

### Table 8.1  Fiber Sources

| Fiber | Source |
| --- | --- |
| Bran | Whole grain products. |
| Pectin | Apples, bananas, beets, cabbage, carrots, citrus fruits, dried peas, okra, and sunflower seeds. |
| Cellulose | Apples, beets, Brazil nuts, broccoli, carrots, green beans, lima beans, pears, peas, and whole grain products. |
| Hemicellulose | Apples, bananas, beans, beets, cabbage, corn, greens, pears, peppers, and whole grain products. |
| Lignin | Brazil nuts, carrots, green beans, peaches, peas, strawberries, tomatoes, and whole grain products. |
| Gums and Mucilages | Dried beans (black, garbonzo, kidney, navy, and pinto), oat bran, oatmeal, peas (black-eyed, lentils, and split), and sesame seeds. |

foods." A plant-based diet, including grains, legumes, vegetables, and fruits, provides optimum dietary fiber.

## WHAT YOU CAN DO ON A PERSONAL LEVEL

To help reduce your odds against some forms of cancer and other illnesses due to lack of dietary fiber, take the following suggestions.

☐ Include 30–40 grams of fiber in your diet each day, especially from complex carbohydrates (foods that contain both starch and fiber). Complex carbohydrates include such foods as whole grain cereals, breads, pasta, potatoes, lentils, chickpeas, and other beans and legumes. Complex carbohydrates are equal in calories (per gram) to protein, and they can help prevent obesity by reducing hunger and giving a feeling of fullness after only a few calories are consumed. As competitive athletes know, complex carbohydrates are also ideal energy foods.

☐ Do not take laxatives for constipation or to cleanse your digestive system. They can irritate the colon and are habit-forming. Fiber supplements that help prevent constipation and move food through the colon quickly include oat and rice bran, glucomannan, guar gum, fennel seed, and psyllium seed. Psyllium seed is contained in Fiberall, Metamucil, and the all-natural fiber supplement Aerobic Bulk Cleanser (ABC), which can be found in most natural foods stores.

## HOW TO GET MORE INVOLVED

It is important to keep abreast of current health-related information. Play an active role in showing your concern.

☐ Support organizations that keep the public informed of important nutritional breakthroughs and other current health information. The following national organizations are actively involved in issues concerning food and nutrition. (Additional information on the organizations is found beginning on page 269.)

Center for Science in the
  Public Interest
Suite 300
1875 Connecticut Avenue, NW
Washington, DC 20009-5728
(202) 332-9110

Community Nutrition
  Institute
Suite 500
2001 S Street, NW
Washington, DC 20009
(202) 462-4700

Public Citizen
2000 P Street, NW
Washington, DC 20036
(202) 833-3000

# Chapter 9

# LACK OF VITAMINS AND MINERALS

There have been major strides in cancer treatment during the last two decades, but very few studies have focused on cancer prevention. Nutrition is the logical area to initiate a preventive approach, because, according to the National Academy of Sciences, up to 60 percent of cancer is related to diet.

It has been widely reported that vitamins A, C, E, and selenium can provide protection against cancer. The B vitamins, calcium together with vitamin D, vitamin K, and copper are also being studied for their beneficial relationship to cancer. In addition, the minerals zinc and magnesium are known to support and help regulate the immune system.

The United States Food and Nutrition Board establishes and periodically re-evaluates Recommended Daily Allowances (RDAs) for each vitamin and mineral based on the amount that is needed to prevent clinical symptoms of nutrient deficiency. However, many doctors, nutritionists, and researchers believe that these RDAs are well below the levels required to achieve and maintain optimal health. For Optimal Daily Allowances (ODAs), see Table 9.1.

## Table 9.1    Optimal Daily Allowances

| Nutrient | Major Uses | Food Sources | RDA | ODA |
|---|---|---|---|---|
| Vitamin A; beta-carotene | Prevents night blindness and other eye problems. May be useful for acne and other skin disorders Enhances immunity. Cancer prevention. May heal gastrointestinal ulcers. Protects against pollution. Needed for epithelial tissue maintenance . | Fish liver oils, animal livers, green and yellow fruits and vegetables | 4,000– 5,000 IU | 10,000–75,000 IU (in a mixture of A and beta-carotene) |
| *B Complex* B-1 (thiamin); B-2 (ribo-flavin); B-3 (niacin, niacinamide) B-6 (pyri-doxine) | Maintains healthy nerves, skin, eyes, hair, liver, mouth, muscle tone in gastrointestinal tract. B vitamins are coenzymes involved in energy production. Emotional or physical stress increases need. May be useful for depression or anxiety. | Unrefined whole grains, liver, green leafy vegetables, fish, poultry, eggs, meat, nuts, beans | 1.2–14 mg | 25–300 mg |

B-1: High-carbohydrate diet increases need.
B-2: May be useful with B-6 for treatment of carpal tunnel syndrome. May prevent cataracts. Increased need with oral contraceptives. Increased need with strenuous exercise.
B-3: Useful for circulatory problems. Lowers serum cholesterol and triglycerides.
B-6: May be useful in preventing oxalate stones. May be used as mild diuretic. May be useful for PMS. Increased need with oral contraceptives. May be useful in treating asthma.

| Nutrient | Major Uses | Food Sources | RDA | ODA |
|---|---|---|---|---|
| B-12 (cobalamin) | Needed for fat and carbohydrate metabolism. Prevention and treatment of B-12 anemia. Maintains proper nervous system function. May be useful for anxiety. | Kidney, liver, egg, herring, mackerel, milk, cheese, tofu, seafood | 2 mcg | 25–300 mcg |
| Vitamin C (ascorbic acid) | Growth and repair of tissues. May reduce cholesterol. Antioxidant. Cancer prevention. Enhances immunity. Stress increases requirement. May reduce high blood pressure. May prevent atherosclerosis. Protects against pollution. | Green vegetables, berries, citrus fruit | 60 mg | 500–5,000 mg (higher during stress or illness) |

| Nutrient | Major Uses | Food Sources | RDA | ODA |
|----------|-----------|--------------|-----|-----|
| Vitamin D | Required for calcium and phosphorus absorption and utilization. Prevention and treatment of osteoporosis. Enhances immunity. | Fish liver oils, fatty saltwater fish. Vitamin D-fortified dairy products, eggs | 400 IU | 400–600 IU |
| Vitamin E | Antioxidant. Cancer prevention. Cardiovascular disease prevention. Improves circulation. Tissue repair. May prevent age spots. Useful in treating fibrocystic breasts. Useful in treating PMS. | Cold-pressed vegetable oils, whole grains, dark-green leafy vegetables, nuts, legumes | 8–10 IU | 200–800 IU |
| Vitamin K | Needed for blood clotting. May play a role in bone formation. May prevent osteoporosis. | Green leafy vegetables | 65–80 mcg | |
| Calcium | Needed for healthy bones and teeth. Needed for nerve transmission. Used for muscle function. May lower blood pressure. Osteoporosis prevention. | Dairy foods, salmon, sardines, green leafy vegetables, seafood | 1,200 mg | 1,000–1,500 mg |
| Copper | Involved in blood formation. Needed for healthy nerves. Needed for taste sensitivity. Used in energy production. Needed for healthy bone development. | Widely distributed in foods, copper cookware, and copper plumbing | None | Needs can generally be met through food: 0.5–2 mg |
| Folic acid | Works closely with B-12. Involved in protein metabolism. Needed for healthy cell division and replication. Prevention and treatment of folic acid anemia. Stress may increase need. May be useful for depression and anxiety. May be useful in treating cervical dysplasia. Oral contraceptives may increase need. | Beef, lamb, pork, chicken liver, green leafy vegetables, whole wheat, bran, yeast | 180–200 mcg | 400–1,200 mcg |

| Nutrient | Major Uses | Food Sources | RDA | ODA |
|----------|-----------|--------------|-----|-----|
| Magnesium | Needed for healthy bones. Involved in nerve transmission. Needed for muscle function. Used in energy formation. Needed for healthy blood vessels. May lower blood pressure. | Widely distributed in foods, especially dairy foods, meat, fish, seafood | 280–350 mg | 500–700 mg |
| Selenium | Cancer prevention. Heart disease prevention. | Depends on soil content, may be in grains and meat | 55–70 mcg | 50–400 mcg (50–100 mcg for those who live in high-selenium areas) |
| Zinc | Needed for wound healing. Maintains taste and smell acuity. Needed for healthy immune system. Protects liver from chemical damage. | Oysters, fish, seafood, meats, poultry, whole grains, legumes | 12–15 mg | 22.5–50 mg |

SOURCE: *The Real Vitamin & Mineral Book* by Shari Lieberman and Nancy Bruning. Garden City Park, NY: Avery Publishing Group, 1990. Adaptation of Quick-Reference Chart.

## A CLOSER LOOK

The following vitamins and minerals are believed to play an important role in cancer prevention.

### Selenium

The adult RDA (Recommended Dietary Allowance) for selenium is 70 micrograms (mcg, or one millionth of a gram) for men and 55 mcg for women; higher amounts could be toxic. Good selenium sources include seafood, beef, pork, lamb, chicken, whole grains, dairy products, eggs, and, depending on the selenium content of the soil, fruits and vegetables.

With vitamins A, C, and E, and the body's own enzymes, selenium is an important *antioxidant*. Antioxidants neutralize *free radicals* (molecular particles containing highly charged, unstable electrons that are the by-products of fat metabolism).

Free radicals are produced when polyunsaturates oxidize, disrupting the chain of oxygen supplies. This creates a chain reaction that damages cells, leaving them vulnerable to the effects of cancer-causing substances. Free radicals are implicated in more than sixty disorders, including cancer, heart disease, Alzheimer's disease, Parkinson's disease, cataracts, and rheumatoid arthritis, as well as an increased susceptibility to auto-immune disorders.

Oxidation takes place when oils are exposed to air or to heat (room temperature heat and/or the high heat used in cooking). Oxidation also takes place inside the body as oils interact with the by-products of cellular metabolism, as well as with radiation, environmental pollutants (smog, tobacco smoke, automobile exhaust), trace metals (copper, nickel, iron), pesticides, and asbestos or other chemical carcinogens.

The antioxidants selenium, vitamin A and beta-carotene, vitamin C, and vitamin E block the cancer initiation process and help preserve the cell's DNA—the genetic material necessary for healthy cell reproduction.

### Vitamin A and Beta-carotene

The adult RDA for vitamin A is 1,000 mcg of RE (retinol equivalent) for men and 800 mcg of RE for women, or 6,000 mcg of beta-carotene for men and 4,800 mcg for women. Higher amounts of vitamin A could be toxic; beta-carotene is non-toxic. Active vitamin A is found only in animal sources, including fish oil (especially oil from cod, halibut, salmon, and shark), beef and chicken liver, and eggs and dairy products. Beta-carotene is found only in green and yellow-orange vegetables and in fruits including carrots, kale, kohlrabi, parsley, spinach, turnip greens, dandelion greens, apricots, and cantaloupe. Beta-carotene converts in the body to usable vitamin A, and it may provide its own protection against cancer in addition to that which is provided by vitamin A. Although it is non-toxic, excessive amounts of beta-carotene can turn the skin yellowish-orange.

With selenium and vitamins C and E, vitamin A and beta-carotene are important antioxidants that can help block the cancer initiation process by neutralizing free radicals. Vitamin A can protect specifically against cancers of the breast, cervix, gastroinestinal tract, larynx, lung, and prostate. It has also been shown that vitamin A protects the lungs against passive (secondhand) cigarette smoke and air pollution. It is, thus, a particularly important nutrient for the 158 million people who live in or near the urban areas that the EPA considers to be unhealthy (see Chapter 19, *Outdoor Hazards*).

### B Vitamins

The B vitamins, many of which are found together in some foods, work synergistically in the body. For this reason, it is important to consume foods or take supplements that contain the entire B complex, including $B_1$ (thiamin), $B_2$ (riboflavin), $B_3$ (niacin and niacinamide), $B_6$ (pyridoxine), $B_{12}$ (cobalamin), folic acid, pantothenic acid, biotin, choline, inositol, and PABA (para-aminobenzoic acid).

* *Folic acid*, or *folate*. The adult RDA is 200 mcg for men and 180 mcg for women. Sources of folic acid include beef, lamb, pork, chicken liver, fruits, berries, melon, bananas, kale, broccoli, asparagus, spinach, beet greens, lima beans, potatoes, eggs, whole wheat, bran, yeast, and peanut butter. Presently, at the Fred Hutchinson Cancer Research Center in Seattle, Washington, folate is being studied for its relationship to the reversal of the precancerous condition known as cervical dysplasia. Folate is also being studied at the University of Alabama as an inhibitor of precancerous bronchial squamous metaplasia (cell change) in smokers.

* *Vitamin $B_2$ (riboflavin)*. The adult RDA is 1.7 mg for men and 1.3 mg for women. Studies have shown that a deficiency of

riboflavin can hamper the immune system's ability to produce antibodies and may increase susceptibility to esophageal cancer. Sources of vitamin $B_2$ include beef, chicken,
dairy products, broccoli, asparagus, beans, leafy green
vegetables, avocados, currants, asparagus, nuts, fish, and
eggs.

- *Vitamin $B_3$ (niacin* and *niacinamide).* The adult RDA is 1.7 mg
  for men and 1.3 mg for women. Sources of vitamin $B_3$
  include lean meats, poultry, fish, whole wheat, potatoes,
  legumes, broccoli, carrots, dairy products, avocados, dates,
  figs, prunes, corn flour, and peanut butter. In its form
  nicotinamide, niacin has been shown in tests at the Eppley
  Institute for Research in Cancer at the University of Ne-
  braska at Omaha to inhibit pancreatic cancer. It is also an
  enzyme cofactor in the production of prostaglandins,
  which regulate tumor growth.

- *Vitamin $B_6$ (pyridoxine).* The adult RDA is 2.0 mg for men
  and 1.6 mg for women. Sources of vitamin $B_6$ include meat,
  poultry, fish (especially herring and salmon), milk, whole
  grains (especially wheat bran and wheat germ), egg yolks,
  potatoes, avocados, kale, spinach, carrots, onions, sweet
  potatoes, lentils, brewer's yeast, walnuts, peas, and bananas. Studies at Oregon State University have shown that
  $B_6$ bolsters the immune system, which, when it is function-
  ing optimally, can kill cancer cells. According to a 1991
  study by the United States Department of Agriculture, too
  little vitamin $B_6$ can lower the immune response, especially
  in older people. Vitamin $B_6$ is also an enzyme cofactor in
  the production of prostaglandins, which regulate tumor
  growth.

- *Vitamin $B_{12}$ (cobalamin).* The adult RDA for both men and
  women is 2 mcg. Sources of vitamin $B_{12}$ include meat
  (especially kidney and liver), pork, tofu, dairy products,
  and seafood (oysters, crabs, clams, herring, mackerel, sardines, tuna). At Memorial Sloan-Kettering Cancer Center in

New York, studies suggest that B12 is needed to help prevent DNA damage, which otherwise can result in damaged cells becoming cancerous. At the University of Alabama, studies are being run to test B12 with folate as a possible inhibitor of precancerous bronchial cells in smokers.

**Vitamin C**

The adult RDA for vitamin C is 60 mg. Vitamin C sources include citrus fruits, melons, berries (vine or tree-ripened for maximum vitamin C content, and refrigerated once picked), black currants, guava, kale, collard greens, parsley, horseradish, green peppers, and cruciferous vegetables (bok choy, broccoli, Brussels sprouts, cabbage, cauliflower, collards, kale, kohlrabi, mustard greens, rutabaga, turnips, and turnip greens).

Vitamin C, a primary antioxidant, also helps prevent the formation of the potent carcinogens known as *nitrosamines.* Nitrosamines are formed when nitrites—found in bacon, sausage, and other pickled, salted or smoked foods react with other chemicals found in food or in the body.

A study done by Gladys Block, Ph.D., at the National Cancer Institute, indicated that people with the highest amounts of vitamin C in their diets have the lowest risk of cancer. Vitamin C is also a catalyst for the formation of prostaglandins, which control tumor growth.

According to research reported in December 1991 in the *Proceedings of the National Academy of Sciences,* levels of vitamin C that are below the recommended daily allowance of 60 milligrams a day may increase the risk of genetic damage to sperm. Genetically damaged sperm can cause birth defects, childhood cancers, and pregnancies that terminate in spontaneous abortion.

According to Geoffrey Howe, Ph.D., Director of Epidemiology of the National Cancer Institute of Canada, "There is a protective factor against cancer in fruits and vegetables, and vitamin C is the most consistent factor. . . . The strongest evidence for vitamin C is with stomach cancer, then [cancer of the] colon, breast and cervix."

### Calcium and Vitamin D

The adult RDA for calcium is 800 mg for men and 1,200 mg for women. The Adult RDA for vitamin D is 5 mcg for both men and women. Calcium sources include dairy products, sardines, salmon, clams, oysters, shrimp, greens (collard, mustard, turnip, kale, spinach), broccoli, soybeans, tofu, and blackstrap molasses. If calcium is taken in a supplement, it should be taken at bedtime; the body needs calcium to repair itself at night, and if calcium is not available, the body draws it from the bones. Also, if calcium supplements or calcium food sources are ingested with fiber foods, the fiber foods bind the calcium, effectively making it nutritionally unavailable.

Vitamin D is obtained by exposure to sunlight, and is found in oily fish (sardines, sea bass, swordfish, cod, herring, tuna, salmon) and in fortified dairy products.

Calcium can decrease the rate of tumor growth in the colon and bowel. Vitamin D enables the body to absorb calcium by helping form a calcium-binding protein in the cells of the intestinal wall; this protein carries calcium through the wall into the bloodstream. Vitamin D protects against colon, bowel, and skin cancer, and leukemia.

### Vitamin E

The adult RDA for vitamin E is 10 mg a-TE (a-Tocopherol) for men and 8 mg a-TE for women. Vitamin E sources include wheat germ, whole wheat and whole wheat products, soybeans, vegetable oils, broccoli, Brussels sprouts, and leafy green vegetables.

An important antioxidant, vitamin E can protect tissue against damage caused by free radicals. Vitamin E also works with vitamin A to protect the lungs from air pollution. It enhances the effect of selenium and can help change cancer cells back to normal cells.

### Vitamin K

The adult RDA for vitamin K is 80 mcg for men and 65 mcg for women. Sources of vitamin K include dark green leafy vegetables, especially sea vegetables (kelp, arame, wakame, nori, kombu, carageenan) that are frequently used in Oriental and macrobiotic cooking.

Studies at the UCLA School of Medicine indicate that in the laboratory, vitamin K—known primarily as a coagulant—kills cancer cells found in the breasts, colon, ovaries, and lungs.

### Copper

There is no established RDA for copper; 2 mg daily is considered a safe dose. Sources of copper include navy beans, whole wheat, avocados, crab meat, nuts and seeds, apricots, bananas, and chicken. Tests performed at the University of Arkansas indicate that copper protects the body against harmful effects of radiation. Studies indicate that copper might be effective in slowing down or or preventing tumor growth.

### Magnesium

The adult RDA for magnesium is 350 mg for men and 280 mg for women. Sources of magnesium include figs, lemons, grapefruit, yellow corn, almonds and other nuts, seeds, dark green leafy vegetables, and apples. Magnesium is an enzyme cofactor necessary for the production of prostaglandins, which control tumor growth.

### Zinc

The adult RDA for zinc is 15 mg for men and 12 mg for women. Doses over 150 mg, however, can be toxic. Too much zinc can impair copper absorption. Sources of zinc include beef, lamb, pork, poultry, seafood (especially oysters),wheat germ, brewer's yeast, eggs, pumpkin seeds, nonfat dry milk, whole grains, peanuts, and ground mustard.

Zinc is an enzyme cofactor that is necessary for the production of prostaglandins, which control tumor growth. Zinc helps regulate the body's immune response, enabling white blood cells—particularly those known as T cells—to kill cancer cells. Researchers at the Howard Hughes Medical Institute of Houston found that adenosine deaminase, an enzyme that sustains immune system function, can act only in the presence of zinc. Zinc also protects against cadmium toxicity. Too much, or, conversely, too little zinc can suppress the immune system.

## WHAT YOU CAN DO ON A PERSONAL LEVEL

Be sure that your diet includes the proper amount of the vitamins and minerals that have been reported to provide protection against cancer (discussed in first section of chapter). Helpful suggestions follow.

☐ Nutrients are best absorbed through whole foods, but be aware that in many regions the soil is seriously depleted of minerals. Much produce is deprived of nutrients because it is harvested too early and stored too long, often without proper refrigeration. Unless your diet is conscientiously balanced, consider a comprehensive vitamin-mineral-trace element supplement to help you maintain your nutritional health.

☐ Buy supplements that contain nutrients derived from natural sources that are formulated in a natural base. Choose supplements without artifical colors or preservatives, including the commonly used antioxidant preservatives BHA (butylated hydroxyanisole) and BHT (butylated hydroxytoluene). Write to the manufacturer of the products that you use and ask for the latest reports on the folowing:

• *Potency.* Tells if the product contains 100 percent of the nutrients listed on the label.
• *Stability.* Shows the expected expiration date.
• *Dissolvability.* Tells if the product passes through the body before it is absorbed.

☐  The following books are excellent sources for further information on the benefits of vitamins and minerals.

*Cancer and Nutrition: A Ten Point Plan to Reduce Your Chances of Getting Cancer* by Charles B. Simone, M.D. Garden City Park, NY: Avery Publishing Group, 1992.

*Prescription for Nutritional Healing* by James F. Balch, M.D., and Phylis Balch, C.N.C. Garden City Park, NY: Avery Publishing Group, 1990.

*The Real Vitamin and Mineral Book* by Shari Lieberman and Nancy Bruning. Garden City Park, NY: Avery Publishing Group, 1990.

*Vitamins Against Cancer* by Redar N. Prasad, Ph.D. Rochester, VT: Healing Arts Press, 1984.

## HOW TO GET MORE INVOLVED

Show your concern on issues that focus attention on food and nutrition.

☐  Actively support organizations that work hard to keep the public aware and informed on important nutritional breakthroughs and other health information. The following national organizations are actively involved on food and nutrition issues. (Additional information on the organizations is found beginning on page 269.)

Center for Science in the
  Public Interest
Suite 300
1875 Connecticut Avenue, NW
Washington, DC 20009-5728
(202) 332-9110

Community Nutrition
  Institute
Suite 500
2001 S Street, NW
Washington, DC 20009
(202) 462-4700

Public Citizen
2000 P Street, NW
Washington, DC 20036
(202) 833-3000

# Chapter 10

# MEAT, POULTRY, AND FISH

The meat we eat today is a far cry from the beef, lamb, and pork our forefathers ate. Today's meat largely comes from animals that have been fed antibiotics, steroids, sex hormones, and pesticide-treated grains since birth. Approximately *one-half* of all antibiotics sold in the United States today are fed to farm animals; together with steroids, antibiotics are used to increase weight and prevent infections. Hormones are also used to promote fast growth and to bring all the animals in a herd into heat at same time for breeding purposes.

Most of the chemicals found in meat are not affected by hot or cold temperatures. Unlike bacteria (some of which can be killed by cooking), these chemicals stay in the animal's flesh no matter how it has been stored or prepared.

Chickens and turkeys are also treated with antibiotics and chemicals in their feed. These toxins accumulate in fatty tissue, livers, and kidneys; they can endanger the health of both the animals themselves and people who eat them.

People who eat fish from United States waterways consume hundreds of toxic substances, including pesticides, mercury, lead, DDT (dichlorodiphenyltrichloroethane), dioxin, chlordane, and PCBs (polychlorinated biphenyls). PCBs have been used as coolants, lubricants and insulating fluids, but they were banned in 1979 when they were linked to cancer. Many PCBs were dumped in wetlands or in landfills that were close to rivers and harbors. With other toxins, such as DDT, PCBs still leak into inland and coastal waters.

Consumers Union reported in 1992 that in a study of fish in retail markets in Chicago and New York, PCBs contaminated almost 43 percent of the salmon, half of the whitefish, and a quarter of the swordfish. In this study, sole and flounder had the lowest levels of PCBs, mercury, and pesticides. Another study found that DDT, which was banned in 1972, continued to show up in 334 of 386 domestic fish samples in 1983.

According to Jeffrey Foran, Ph.D., of George Washington University's Division of Occupational and Environmental Medicine, people who eat small amounts of salmon, lake trout, and other chemically contaminated sports fish have a higher cancer risk. Many states have issued recommendations on how much fish to eat. In Wisconsin—depending on the body of water from which fish are taken—the State Department of Natural Resources, Division of Health, divides contaminated fish into three groups: fish that everyone can eat in restricted quantities, fish that children and pregnant or nursing women should not eat, and fish that no one should ever eat at all. (From Lake Michigan, for instance, no one should ever eat trout that is over 23 inches long, chinook salmon that is over 32 inches long, brown trout over 23 inches in length, carp, or catfish.)

Some of New York's waterways have been closed entirely to commercial and sport fishing. New York's Department of Health recommends that people eat no more than one-half pound of fish a week from New York waters. Nursing and pregnant women should avoid all New York State freshwater fish, and everyone should avoid striped bass taken from Long Island waters west of Wading River. (Striped bass from eastern Long Island can be eaten once a month.)

High levels of mercury, which affects the development of the nervous system, and DDT have been found in fish from California waters (especially swordfish, tuna, halibut, walleye, and red snapper). Fish caught in the Fox River on Chicago's outskirts and in Washington's Puget Sound have themselves been found to have a high incidence of cancer. Never eat fish caught from these places, or those from New York's Hudson River, Ohio's Black River, Boston Harbor, or Ontario's Hamilton Harbor.

According to the Center for Science in the Public Interest (CSPI), approximately 12 percent of the fish eaten in the United States today are farm raised. In this process, known as *aquaculture*, fish are bred, raised, and harvested under environmentally controlled conditions. Some farmed fish, especially catfish, have developed antibiotic-resistant strains of bacteria that can be transferred to humans.

Farm-raised fish that are reared in small, confined spaces are often treated with drugs to control stress-related diseases. Some of the drugs used in fish farming have been in use for many years and may be legal for use in other animal species, but most of these drugs have not been approved by the FDA for use in aquaculture. Furthermore, the drugs may not be withdrawn from the fish in time to pass out of their bodies before they are sold and eaten.

The farmed fish that you buy may have been fed illegal color additives to tint their flesh. Because of the type of feed used, these fish may also have lower levels of the beneficial omega-3 fatty acids that are found in wild fish (see Chapter 5, *Dietary Fat*).

High heat used in grilling, frying, or broiling meat, poultry, and fish can form cancer-causing heterocyclic aromatic amines (HHAs). The higher the heat and the longer the cooking time, the greater the amount of HHAs produced. Baking and roasting produce fewer HHAs, and stewing, boiling, poaching, and microwaving produce almost none.

Organic meat (from animals that have not been treated with any chemicals and that have been fed natural grains) is available in natural foods stores and in some supermarkets. In general, however, meat tends to be high in fat, and a high-fat diet in itself has been implicated in a number of cancers (see Chapter 5, *Dietary Fat*).

## WHAT YOU CAN DO ON A PERSONAL LEVEL

Lowering possible cancer risks from eating meat, poultry, and fish requires a few simple lifestyle changes.

☐ Eat less meat, poultry, and fish. When you do eat these foods, be sure to remove all fat, because pesticides and other toxins accumulate in fatty tissue.

☐ Buy organic beef and chicken.

☐ Do not eat liver, kidneys, or sweetbreads, because toxic substances accumulate in organ meats.

☐ Use non-fat (skim) milk, because pesticides and other chemicals ingested by cows can be found in milk fat.

☐ Keep informed of pollution problems in your local fishing waters. Call your State Department of Health and ask them to send you current recommendations for eating fish from bodies of water in your state.

☐ Do not eat coastal or freshwater fish, including salmon, herring, or sardines. Eat fish that are low in fat and that live in deep waters far out at sea. The safest offshore fish to eat are cod, scrod, flounder, haddock, pollock, sole, and yellowfin tuna. The next safest fish are hake, halibut, ocean perch, pompano, albacore tuna, and tilefish.

☐ Do not eat the following fish: bass; swordfish; bluefish; yellow or white perch; rainbow, brook, or lake trout; whitefish; catfish; or carp.

☐ Buy smaller (younger) fish; they accumulate fewer toxins in their shorter lifetimes.

☐ After cooking fish, trim away the dark meat and the tail, which are the fattiest tissues.

☐ Cook with low heat. Do not charcoal grill beef, poultry, or fish. When grilling, fat drips onto the flame, resulting in smoke that rises and saturates the food with toxic substances, including the potent carcinogen *pyrobenzene*. Grilled food also absorbs dangerous chemicals, which are released from charcoal briquettes.

☐ To grill meat, poultry, or fish, wrap and seal the food in foil before cooking it, or place foil that has been punctured with holes, below the food. This will allow the fat to drip through the foil while protecting the food from flame flare-ups and smoke. The safest method of grilling is with the flame above the food.

☐ Consider a vegetarian or a vegan vegetarian (no meat, poultry, fish, or dairy products) diet. Combine grains and legumes (beans) or use soy products for protein.

☐ Consult the following books for further information on vegetarian diets:

*Diet for a Small Planet* by Frances Moore Lappe. New York: Ballantine Books, 1971.

*Food and Healing* by Annemarie Colbin. New York: Ballantine Books, 1986.

*The Macrobiotic Approach to Cancer* by Michio Kushi. Garden City Park, NY: Avery Publishing Group, 1988.

*The Macrobiotic Cancer Prevention Cookbook* by Aveline Kushi and Wendy Esko. Garden City Park, NY: Avery Publishing Group, 1988.

*Macrobiotics and Beyond* by Marcea and Daniel Weber. Garden City Park, NY: Avery Publishing Group, 1988.

*Making the Transition to a Macrobiotic Diet* by Carolyn Heidenry. Garden City Park, NY: Avery Publishing Group, 1987.

*The Vegetarian Epicure* by Anna Thomas. New York: Vintage Books, 1972.

*The Vegetarian Epicure, Book Two* by Anna Thomas. New York: Alfred A. Knopf, 1987.

## HOW TO GET MORE INVOLVED

If you are concerned with issues on food safety and nutrition, there are avenues that you can take to become more actively involved.

☐ Ask your grocery store owner or manager to carry at least a small selection of meats and poultry that have been organically grown.

☐ Support organizations that have been established to inform and protect citizens on matters concerning food safety and nutrition. The following are a few of such worthwhile organizations. (Additional information on the groups is found beginning on page 269.)

Center for Science in the
    Public Interest
Suite 300
1875 Connecticut Avenue
Washington, DC 20009-5728
(202) 332-9110

Community Nutrition
    Institute
Suite 500
2000 S Street, NW
Washington, DC 20009
(202) 462-4700

Public Citizen
2000 P Street, NW
Washington, DC 20036
(202) 833-3000

# Chapter 11

# PESTICIDES IN FOOD

Pesticides are used on food crops to control weeds, insects, fungi, and rodents. Pesticide use increases crop yields, lengthens shelf life, and improves the appearance of fruits, vegetables, and grains. Food producers use ten times more pesticides today than when they were first introduced in the 1940s. Pesticides are found in virtually all kinds of foods, including meat, poultry, fish, dairy products, vegetables, fruit, coffee, sugar, cooking oil, cereals, canned goods, pet food, rice, and other grains. Unless we eat organic food that has been grown in pesticide-free soil, we consume pesticides every day. Pesticides are also found in the water that we drink and cook with (see *Water*, Chapter 25).

Presently, over 600 chemical pesticides are on the market, distributed in an estimated 35,000 to 50,000 mixtures. Of the 320 pesticides approved for use on food crops, the Environmental Protection Agency (EPA) acknowledges that at least 66 are suspected carcinogens. Consumer-protection organizations believe this estimate is low. Pesticides are mixed with over 1,200 "inert" ingredients, which have no pest-killing action, but that can include the known carcinogens methylene chloride, benzene, and xylene. Because formulas are considered "trade secrets," manufacturers don't have to list inert ingredients on their labels.

According to the Sierra Club publication *Pesticide Alert: A Guide to Pesticides in Fruits and Vegetables* by Lawrie Mott and

Karen Snyder, of the 2½ billion pounds of pesticides that are used in the United States each year, 60 percent are used in agriculture, largely to keep food looking better longer. Many pesticides cause cancer and birth defects (90 percent of mutagens—sources of birth defects—cause cancer as well), and many more are suspected carcinogens that have not yet been tested.

Some pesticides, such as parathion, are so potent that a few drops can cause death on contact. The EPA has banned many pesticides that have been linked to birth defects, genetic defects, and cancer, but these toxic substances continue to turn up in our food and water supplies. Dichlorodiphenyltrichloroethane (DDT), aldrin, and endrin—banned for agricultural use in the 1970s—are still used for other purposes. The EPA continues to permit the use of aldrin as a termiticide, and individual states can petition the EPA to use DDT and endrin if an agricultural infestation problem does not respond to other pesticides. A Natural Resources Defense Council (NRDC) survey found that these pesticides still appear in our fruits, vegetables, and water.

Other pesticides that are banned for use in the United States are produced by American manufacturers for export to other countries. These pesticides often return to us in imported foods, especially coffee, chocolate, rice, tea, sugar, tapioca, and bananas and other fruits.

Little is known about how different pesticides interact with each other and with other chemicals, because the potential combinations are too numerous to study. Many environmental scientists and consumer-protection organizations believe that combinations of carcinogenic substances produce higher toxic levels than any single chemical compound would produce if used alone.

Pesticides have made front-page news in the last decade. In 1985, over 1,000 people in the western United States and Canada were poisoned by watermelon that contained the pesticide Temik, a brand of aldicarb. Reported symptoms included gastrointestinal disorders, blurred vision, muscle weakness, grand mal seizures, cardiac irregularities, and stillbirths.

In 1986, approximately 140 dairy herds in Arkansas, Oklahoma, and Missouri were quarantined due to contamination by the pesticide heptachlor, which was banned in 1976; these herds had ingested heptachlor in livestock feed, which the manufacturer knew was contaminated when it was sold to dairy farmers. Some of the milk that was produced contained seven times the acceptable heptachlor level as established by the EPA.

In 1989, consumers responded so forcefully to an NRDC report on the risk to children from pesticides—in particular from *Alar* (daminozide) in apples—that many supermarkets agreed not to sell Alar-treated apples or apple products. Alar is a systemic pesticide that cannot be removed by washing or peeling. Systemic chemicals are absorbed by the tree or plant, and flow inside the fruit. Government and industry officials tried to reassure the public that so few growers used Alar that risk was minimal, but independent testing by Consumers Union refuted their claims.

Finally, five years after acknowledging that Alar might cause cancer, and that if it remained in use nearly 11,000 additional cancer deaths could result by the year 2033, the EPA banned Alar. (If either the maker or users of a pesticide should protest an EPA ban, the product can remain on the market for several years until the appeal is resolved.)

Pesticides can cause sickness or even death to farm workers who apply them. A National Cancer Institute (NCI) study found that farmers in Kansas who were exposed to herbicides more than twenty days a year, were six times more likely to contract lymphatic cancer.

In 1988, Cesar Chavez, president of the United Farm Workers, was joined by environmental, consumer, and public health groups in supporting a union boycott of pesticide-sprayed grapes. Chavez called for a ban on the pesticides that were considered to be most dangerous: captan, dinoseb, methyl bromide, parathion, and Phosdrin. Growers contended that all five of these chemicals were safe "when used properly." In the fall of 1991, after a consortium of environmental groups jointly petitioned the EPA, parathion was banned for use on all hand-harvested crops, including grapes. (The other chemicals on Chavez' list are still in use.)

NRDC reported in its 1988 publication *Intolerable Risk: Pesticides in Our Children's Food* that between 5,500 and 6,200 current American preschoolers under the age of six may eventually get cancer as a result of exposure to eight commonly used pesticides. Children are more susceptible than adults because they consume fruits, especially apples and apple products, in far greater quantities than adults do.

The EPA and the Food and Drug Administration (FDA) are jointly responsible for protecting the public from pesticide residues. The EPA, under the Federal Insecticide, Fungicide and Rodenticide Act (FIFRA), regulates the sale and use of pesticides; the FDA enforces food-policy laws, to insure that the food we eat is safe. Using test results provided by the pesticide manufacturers themselves, the EPA determines whether or not a chemical causes "unreasonable adverse effects" on the environment or in humans. If it is determined that benefits outweigh risks (i.e only a small number of deaths will occur), the EPA registers the product and sets a tolerance level (a maximum amount allowed). This tolerance level is based on how much of a particular food that the average, 160-pound adult American male eats (or ate in the 1960s, when tolerance levels were established). For example, the EPA estimates that each year an adult American male eats no more than 7.5 ounces of artichokes, blueberries, cantaloupe, eggplant, filberts, figs, garlic, leeks, mushrooms, nectarines, parsley, papaya, pecans, plums, radishes, rye flour, summer squash, tangerines, or walnuts. People who eat more than half a pound a year of any of these foods may be exposed to a toxic level of pesticide residue.

Tolerance levels do not take into account one's personal, regional, or ethnic dietary habits; the synergistic effect of combining chemicals; the transformation of chemicals during cooking or digestion; widespread changes in eating habits in the last thirty years; or the eating habits of children. The 1988 NRDC report *For Our Kids' Sake* notes that FDA labs can detect only about 40 percent of the chemicals present in food, and most foods are not tested at all. According to the General Accounting Office (GAO), testing procedures in 60 percent of domestic and 45 percent of imported food samples are so slow that before results are in, the food has already been bought and eaten.

In *Pesticide Alert*, Mott and Snyder point out that EPA has, in some cases, licensed products and established tolerances even before tests were completed; and tolerance levels were based on incomplete, invalid, or inaccurate data. Officials of Industrial Bio-Test (IBT) of Northbrook, Illinois—whose data the government originally used to approve pesticides—were convicted in 1983 of fabricating research for both government and industry. (Decisions based on IBT data were later revised.)

Jay Feldman, national coordinator of the National Coalition Against the Misuse of Pesticides (NCAMP), calls FIFRA "the weakest environmental law on the books today." One of FIFRA's provisions gives the EPA the authority to grant emergency requests from users to apply unregistered pesticides, and/or to use pesticides in ways not permitted by their registration. The political activist organization Common Cause reported that from October 1972 to June 1987, 1,348 out of 1,885 of these emergency requests were granted.

When the United States Department of Agriculture (USDA) turned over pesticide regulation to the EPA in 1970, most of the chemicals then in use were simply "grandfathered" into approval with no testing at all. A 1972 FIFRA amendment allowed the continued use of approximately 600 ingredients in 50,000 products on the condition that they be tested in the future for carcinogenic, mutagenic, and teratogenic effects. By 1990, the EPA had evaluated the safety of a handful of these chemicals.

Meanwhile, an increasing number of insects (447 species), weeds, fungi, and rodents have become resistant to the chemicals now used. This has prompted growers to use increased amounts of pesticides and has caused chemical companies to develop newer and even stronger mixtures. In 1945, pest contamination caused 31 percent of crops to fail; in 1988, the failure of 37 percent of crops was due to pests. This statistic obviously gives rise to questions concerning the effectiveness of pesticide use.

## WHAT YOU CAN DO ON A PERSONAL LEVEL

Take the following suggestions, which will help protect you from harmful pesticides commonly found in and on foods.

☐ Remove the outer leaves of leafy vegetables such as cabbage and lettuce; they often contain over thirty times the amount of pesticide residue as the inner leaves.

☐ Wash produce in liquid detergent and warm water. This can remove about 40 percent of surface pesticide residue.

☐ Rinse meat, poultry, fish, eggs, vegetables, and fruit for five minutes in a mixture of ¼ cup of vinegar and 1 gallon of water. The vinegar's acidity catalyzes the breakdown of some pesticides.

☐ If you are sensitized (allergic) to pesticides, and do not have a source for organically grown meat and produce, soak meat, poultry, fish, eggs, vegetables, and fruit in a mixture of ½ teaspoon of Clorox and 1 gallon of filtered or pure spring water. Use only Clorox brand bleach. Soak leafy vegetables, thin-skinned root or fibrous vegetables, and thick-skinned fruit for thirty minutes; soak other vegetables, thin-skinned fruit, fish, meat, poultry, and eggs for twenty minutes. After soaking in the Clorox solution, immerse the food for ten minutes in clear water. For many years, the United States Department of State has recommended this formula to families living in China, Southeast Asia, Turkey, and other countries. In addition to removing surface pesticides, this soaking method can remove bacteria, fungi, parasites, heavy metals, and viruses (including salmonella). Food treated this way before it is stored stays fresh more than twice as long as usual. However, this method should be used only if you are sensitized to pesticides, because chlorine bleach disposed of through household drains can contaminate local water supplies. And use filtered or spring water only; otherwise, organic residue in the water can combine with chlorine to form cancer-causing trihalomethane gases. (See Chapter 25, *Water*.)

☐ Scrub or peel fruits and vegetables, especially root vegetables. Always peel waxed fruits and vegetables, because many waxes contain fungicides, which are used to make food look better and to prevent shriveling and rotting. Apples, avocados, cantaloupes, cucumbers, eggplants, grapefruits, lemons, limes, nectarines, peaches, peppers, sweet potatoes, and tomatoes are frequently waxed.

☐ If possible, buy organically grown foods.

☐ Do not eat imported foods. They may contain banned or unregulated chemicals.

☐ Eat foods that are high in fiber. Dietary fiber can help eliminate some pesticide residues from the body (see Chapter 8, *Lack of Dietary Fiber*).

☐ Eat foods or take supplements that contain antioxidants. Vitamin A, C, E, beta-carotene, and selenium can help detoxify pesticides (see Chapter 9, *Lack of Vitamins and Minerals*).

## HOW TO GET MORE INVOLVED

Speak out against the use of dangerous pesticides on food crops. There are many things that you can do to have your voice heard.

☐ Ask your grocery store owner or manager to stock organically grown foods. Urge that the sale of chemically treated meats, poultry, and produce be discontinued.

☐ Write to your state and federal officials and urge them to do the following:

• ban carcinogenic pesticides.
• require that all pesticides used in food be labeled.
• limit and regulate all pesticides.
• support research on organic growing methods.
• develop alternative methods of growing, preserving, and storing food.

- encourage less toxic existing methods, including Integrated Pest Management (IPM), a system that uses microbes and insect predators. IPM relies on chemicals only when careful monitoring reveals that pests are actually present.

☐ Write to your legislators and demand that standards be developed for certifying organic foods. Maine, California, and several other states have already developed these standards.

☐ For more information, contact any of the following organizations. Support these public-interest groups that pressure legislators to ban or regulate pesticide use on food crops. (Additional information on the organizations is found beginning on page 269.)

Americans for Safe Food
PO Box 66330
Washington, DC 20035
(202) 332-9110

Mothers and Others
  for a Livable Planet
40 West 20th Street
New York, NY 10011
(212) 727-4474

National Coalition Against
  the Misuse of Pesticides
701 E Street, SE – Suite 200
Washington, DC 20003
(202) 543-5450

Natural Resources
  Defense Council
40 West 20th Street
New York, NY 10011
(212) 727-2700

Northwest Coalition for
  Alternatives to Pesticides
PO Box 1393
Eugene, OR 97440
(503) 344-5044

# HOME AND ENVIRONMENT

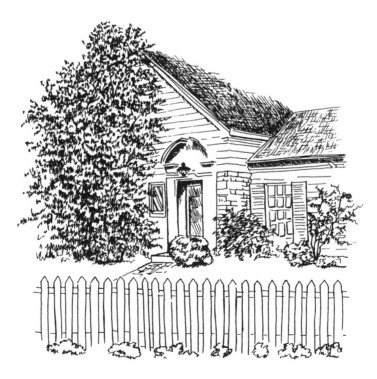

# Chapter 12

# ASBESTOS

Asbestos is the name for a group of natural minerals that separate into strong, very fine fibers. Asbestos has been used in the United States since 1880; its peak use period was from the 1930s through the 1970s.

There are several types of asbestos (lactinolite, amosite, anthophyllite, chrysotile, crocidolite, and tremolite), each named for the mineral it comes from. Nearly 95 percent of asbestos used in the United States today is chrysotile.

Because of asbestos' acid-resistance, tensile strength, light weight, imperviousness to chemicals and heat, and inability to conduct electricity, it has been used in nearly 3,000 products. Some of these products include insulation for heating, water, and sewage pipes; electrical insulation; brake linings; sound absorption and flameproofing materials; roof, siding, and floor tiles; gutter pipes; corrugated paper; filters for liquids; textiles (blankets, sheets, curtains, clothing); paints and coatings; vinyl wallpaper; cement; caulking; putty; and spackle. Asbestos might be found in water that runs through asbestos cement pipes, and in some products containing talc, such as body powder, feminine deodorants, and scouring powder.

Asbestos is friable, which means it crumbles easily. If bonded in finished products, it poses no health risk. However, if the bond is disturbed by sanding, sawing, drilling, or corrosion, the resulting airborne asbestos fibers can be inhaled or swallowed.

Each microscopic asbestos fiber is so fine that it is less than one-hundredth the size of a strand of human hair. If asbestos is inhaled or swallowed, it can remain in the lungs forever, ultimately causing lung cancer or asbestosis. Cases have been reported of workers who brought asbestos dust home on their clothes or their bodies, and fatally exposed family members.

The Environmental Protection Agency (EPA) reported in March 1988 that more than 500,000 office buildings, apartment houses, stores, and other public and commercial buildings contained deteriorating asbestos. Due to the fact that so many school buildings contained asbestos, Congress passed the Asbestos School Hazard Abatement Act in 1984, which provided financial and technical aid for the safe removal of asbestos. Asbestos cement also contaminates an estimated 400,000 miles of water pipes in the United States. Dangerous asbestos levels in water were found in areas as diverse as Bishopville, South Carolina; San Francisco, California; Detroit, Michigan; and Woodstock, New York. In Woodstock, residents were warned not to drink, bathe in, or cook with household water.

The world's foremost asbestos-related disease expert, Irving J. Selikoff, M.D., of the Mt. Sinai School of Medicine in New York, says that asbestos is so potent a carcinogen that a worker who inhales fibers under conditions of heavy exposure for just one day might, as a result, contract lung cancer twenty years later.

The most common source of asbestos is in the insulation wrapped around basement pipes, which, as it deteriorates, may crumble, dusting the floor with a fine light-colored powder.

To treat asbestos in a basement or any other room, trained workers wearing protective jumpsuits and respirators seal the area, then mist the asbestos material to hold down the dangerous dust. The asbestos material and dust is then placed in hazardous waste bags. Next, the pipes are washed, then sealed to trap any remaining fibers; a specially-equipped filtered vacuum is used to remove residue from every crevice and surface. Finally, the sealed refuse is disposed of in a designated hazardous-waste site.

To verify that the air is safe, the contractor takes an air sample. The reading should indicate an asbestos level at or below .01 fibers per cubic centimeter of air—the normal, outdoor level. (Levels are higher in cities such as New York, where there is a great deal of ongoing demolition.)

## WHAT YOU CAN DO ON A PERSONAL LEVEL

Reduce any risk from airborne asbestos by taking the following suggestions.

□ If you suspect there is asbestos insulation in your home, contact a certified asbestos abatement contractor. It is extremely dangerous to allow asbestos to be disturbed by workmen who are uninformed about the hazards or unequipped to protect both themselves and you.

□ If the asbestos insulating material on your pipes, wiring, furnace, or appliances is intact, it can simply be wrapped, sealed, and enclosed in a protective coating. If it is torn and crumbling (usually into a gray-white dust), removal—which might prove to be quite costly—is essential.

□ To locate a certified contractor, or for more information on asbestos inspection, encapsulation, removal, or disposal, contact one of the following resources:

Center for Environmental
  Management
(617) 381-3531

Consumer Product
  Safety Commission
(800) 638-CPSC

EPA
Public Information
(202) 260-2080

Toxic Substances Control
Assistance Information
(202) 554-1404

White Lung Association
(410) 243-5864

☐ If you suspect there is asbestos in your household water, have your water tested by a certified lab. For a list of water-testing laboratories, see page 202.

☐ If necessary, consider installing a water filter to remove asbestos from household water. Information on water-filter systems is found in Chapter 25.

☐ Use cornstarch instead of talc, which may contain asbestos. (Talc-free body powders are available in natural foods stores.)

☐ Use baking soda or borax instead of scouring powders, which may contain asbestos.

☐ A free copy of *Asbestos in Your Home* is available either by writing to or calling:

Publication Request                    EPA Public Information
Consumer Product Safety                401 M Street, SW
   Commission                          Washington, DC 20460
Washington, DC 20207                   (202) 260-2080


HOW TO GET MORE INVOLVED

Consider the following suggestions on lowering risks from asbestos.

☐ Contact your water utility and find out the type of pipes that are used in your municipality. If you discover there is asbestos in your water pipes, ask your neighbors to join you in pressuring your local government to replace all the pipes in the system.

☐ Support the following organizations whose goals are to maintain (among other issues) indoor air quality as it relates to asbestos. (Additional information on the organizations is found beginning on page 269.)

National Center for
  Environmental Health
  Strategies
1100 Rural Avenue
Voorhees, NJ 08043
(609) 429-5358

Safe Buildings Alliance
Metropolitan Square
Suite 1200
655 15th Street, NW
Washington, DC 20005
(202) 879-5120

# Chapter 13

# FORMALDEHYDE

Formaldehyde is a colorless gas that can be emitted from various building materials, household products, and combustion processes. Formaldehyde is used in a wide variety of products either as a solvent, a softener, or as an intermediate in organic synthesis. An intermediate is an organic compound that acts as a bridge between a parent compound and the final product. Organic compounds are used in the production of dyes, pharmaceuticals, and other products that develop properties upon oxidation, such as a hair dye that becomes active only when it is exposed to oxygen.

The most significant formaldehyde sources in homes are pressed-wood products that are made with adhesives containing urea-formaldehyde (UF) resins. These products include particleboard (used as subflooring and for shelving in cabinetry and furniture), hardwood plywood paneling (used in cabinets, furniture, and as decorative wall coverings), and especially medium-density fiberboard (used for drawer fronts, cabinet doors, and furniture tops). Other common formaldehyde sources include curtains, carpets, upholstery fabrics, linens, clothing, and other permanent-press fabrics; urea-formaldehyde foam insulation (UFFI), which was used in the construction and extra insulation of many homes, schools, and other buildings in the 1970s; glues, adhesives, paints, coatings, and cosmetics; and unvented fuel-burning appliances, such as gas stoves and kerosene space heaters.

Formaldehyde is used in the construction of many mobile and prefabricated homes. The interior spaces in these homes are relatively small. Consequently, since 1985, the United States Department of Housing and Urban Development (HUD) has permitted the use of plywood and particleboard in these homes only if the materials conform to specified emission limits.

Soft plywood and other pressed-wood products that are produced for use in exterior construction contain the dark or reddish-black colored phenol-formaldehyde (PF) resin. PF resin usually emits formaldehyde at a much lower rate than UF resin.

New products generally emit the most formaldehyde, especially in conditions of high indoor temperatures and humidity. Emissions decrease as products age. UFFI insulation installed in the 1970s probably no longer emits significant amounts of formaldehyde unless it is damp and/or there are cracks or openings in interior walls that expose the foam.

Eye makeups, perfumes, toothpastes, hairsprays, nail polishes and hardeners, soaps, toilet tissue, disinfectants, and fungicides commonly contain formaldehyde. According to the l938 Food, Drug and Cosmetic Act, formaldehyde has to be labeled if it is used in cosmetics.

Approximately 5.7 billion pounds of formaldehyde are produced each year. Building materials that contain formaldehyde are labeled, but caution tags often fall off. Sometimes the caution tags are removed at the lumberyard or before the materials are delivered. If formaldehyde is present in building materials or insulation, there will be a noticeably strong and pungent odor when these products are first installed.

Formaldehyde emissions, known as off-gassing, cause cancer in animals and are, therefore, suspected of causing cancer in humans. Formaldehyde can produce severe physical reactions, including cold-like symptoms, intense mucous membrane irritation in the nose and throat, burning eyes, nausea, headaches, dizziness, and shortness of breath. High concentrations can trigger asthma attacks. Symptoms can appear immediately or not until months after exposure. Formaldehyde is so potent that if one ounce is ingested, coma and death can result within hours.

## WHAT YOU CAN DO ON A PERSONAL LEVEL

If you suspect that your surroundings have harmful formaldehyde emissions, heed the following suggestions.

☐ If a member of your household experiences symptoms such as those described on page 90, but finds that the symptoms disappear after leaving home for several days, have your home formaldehyde level measured. Detection devices (ranging in price from $25.00–60.00) are available from your local health department, or can be ordered from:

The Ecology Box
260 South Main Street
Ann Arbor, MI 48103
(800) 735-1371
(313) 662-9131

Nontoxic Environments
6135 NW Mountain
  View Drive
Corvallis, OR 97330
(503) 745-7838

Environmental Testing
  & Technology
PO Box 369
Encinitas, CA 92024
(619) 436-5990

Safe Environments
2512 Ninth Street
Berkeley, CA 94710
(800) 356-2663
(510) 549-9693

☐ A formaldehyde problem can usually be solved by removing or sealing the source, and/or through proper ventilation. Your local health department can recommend a remediation specialist.

☐ Ask questions when buying building materials, especially particleboard or prefinished paneling. Find out if the materials have been treated with formaldehyde.

☐ Coat all surfaces and edges of pressed-wood products with polyurethane. This will help reduce formaldehyde emissions. Be sure to buy a coating product that does not contain formaldehyde.

92 *Everyday Cancer Risks and How to Avoid Them*

☐ Maintain adequate ventilation and moderate temperature and humidity levels in the home. Dehumidifiers and air conditioners can help reduce emissions. Vent all fuel-burning appliances. Always cross-ventilate rooms with unvented heaters.

☐ Choose natural-fiber curtains, rugs, carpets, and linoleum. Natural-fiber products are available at large import stores such as Pier 1, Ikea, and Cost Plus. They can also be ordered from:

Collins and Aikman
PO Box 1447
Dalton, GA 30772
(404) 259-9711

Hendricksen Floorcovering
8031 Mill Station Road
Sebastopol, CA 95472
(707) 829-3959

Dellinger
PO Drawer 273
Rome, GA 30161
(404) 291-4447

Sinan Company
PO Box 857
Davis, CA 95617
(916) 753-3104

☐ Always wash wrinkle-resistant clothing and fabrics before wearing or using them. By eliminating some of the formaldehyde through washing, you can help prevent the possible development of flu-like or other physical symptoms.

☐ Table 16.1, beginning on page 118, lists formaldehyde-free household products. Chapter 28, *Cosmetics and Personal-Care Products*, provides information on cosmetics that are formaldehyde free.

☐ If your home has urea-formaldehyde foam insulation, removal can be costly because inner walls may have to be torn down. Contact the following organization for advice on how to approach installers and producers to pay these costs:

CURE Formaldehyde Poisoning Association
Attention: Connie Smrecek
Waconia, MN 55387
(612) 442-4665

☐ If you are a victim of formaldehyde poisoning, help is available. The Formaldehyde Litigation Group can help you with procedural assistance. They will also refer you to a lawyer who is experienced in representing victims of formaldehyde poisoning.

Formaldehyde Litigation Group
622 Drayton Street
Savannah, GA 31401
(800) 222-TORT

**HOW TO GET MORE INVOLVED**

If you are worried about the dangers of formaldehyde emissions, show your concern.

☐ Support organizations that have been established to keep the public informed on the political, medical, and legal issues surrounding formaldehyde. (Additional information on the organizations is found beginning on page 269.)

CURE Formaldehyde
  Poisoning Association
9255 Lynnwood Road
Waconia, MN 55387
(612) 442-4665

National Center for
  Environmental Health
  Strategies
1100 Rural Avenue
Voorhees, NJ 08043
(609) 429-5358

# Chapter 14

# GARBAGE

Americans are generating more garbage than ever before. Municipal solid waste has increased by 80 percent since 1960, and the Environmental Protection Agency (EPA) estimates another 20 percent increase in the next ten years.

According to INFORM, Inc., a natural resources and public-health research organization in New York City, the United States produces about 400,000 tons of solid waste each day (nearly four pounds per person)! This is more garbage than any other industrialized country using comparable consumer goods generates.

Many communities dispose of garbage in landfills and/or incinerators. Most landfills leach a large number of potent carcinogens into our water supplies, while incinerators spew them into our air.

In landfills solid waste is usually buried between layers of earth. Organic garbage is mixed with toxic and caustic chemicals that have been thrown away (e.g. discarded motor oils, paints, household cleaners, metal cans, record albums, batteries, rubber products, and small appliances). Chemicals in these items—many of them cancer-causing substances—form a percolating, toxic liquid known as *leachate*. Gravity pulls leachate down through the soil into the groundwater and any nearby surface water. Rainwater hastens the process by seeping down through the landfill. The water then flows out of the landfill's bottom layer, carrying leached toxins—especially the carcinogens lead and cadmium—into our water supplies.

Within the next decade, most major American cities will run out of landfill space and one-third of America's landfills will be closed. As landfill space dwindles, some municipalities are considering incineration as an alternative. In the incineration process, a complex variety of unsorted garbage is burned, and a variety of toxic airborne pollutants is produced. Over 700 of these toxins have already been identified, including antimony, arsenic, beryllium, cadmium, carbon dioxide, lead, nitrogen, and mercury. Other toxic pollutants being spewed into the atmosphere by incinerators include acid gases, such as hydrogen chloride and fluoride; a variety of chlorinated and brominated compounds, including over seventy-five possible chlorinated dioxins and chlorinated dibenzofurans; and sulfur dioxide, a major component of *acid rain*. Acid rain is the name commonly given to rain or snow that carries destructive chemical compounds. These compounds rise into the air from coal-fired power plants, incinerators, and other industrial sources. They are driven by the wind through the atmosphere, often winding up as far as a thousand miles away, where they fall to earth as acidic rain, snow, fog, or dry particles.

In research conducted in Europe, dioxins and other trace-level toxins that were believed to have been emitted by European incinerators have been found in breastmilk, commercial dairy products, fish, soil, and dust. As a result, Sweden and Denmark instituted a moratorium on incineration plant construction.

In the United States, the Minnesota Pollution Control Agency has concluded that 80 percent of the mercury in Minnesota's lakes comes from the air. Clean Water Action reports that the Semass incinerator in Rochester, Massachusetts, emits 2,000 tons of toxic chemicals every year, including 590 pounds of mercury and 1 ton of lead. These toxins have been linked to cancers of the lung, stomach, large intestine, liver, prostate, and bladder, as well as skin cancer and genetic mutations. Garbage incineration is the fastest-growing source of atmospheric mercury.

Incineration reduces the volume of garbage by 75 to 90 percent; however, it produces toxic ash, both fly ash (collected from the pollution control systems), and bottom ash (collected from the furnace grates). Every year, 5.3 million tons of this toxic residue are transported and dumped into landfills, where rainwater seeps through and carries it into local water systems.

Advocates of incineration have proposed mixing the toxic ash into construction blocks, roadbed materials, landfill covers, and artificial reefs. In December 1990, The nation's first building—a boathouse—containing masonry blocks (cinder blocks) made with incinerator ash was completed and now stands on the State University of New York (SUNY) at Stony Brook campus. The EPA provided funds for SUNY to monitor the surrounding air and soil for toxic emissions from the boathouse for several years. The Waste Management Institute of the Marine Sciences Research Center at SUNY has also built a reef made from incinerator-ash blocks in the Long Island Sound, and it has approved plans for the construction of an incinerator-ash-block seawall. However, the long-term effects of using these building materials are, at present, a matter of conjecture; whether they can withstand the test of generations of use without endangering health is yet unclear.

Incinerators have been implicated so strongly as causes of air pollution and acid rain that many communities are refusing to accept them. One thing everyone agrees on is that we need to develop an innovative approach to waste management that includes source reduction (not generating so much garbage to begin with) as well as recycling. Eighty percent of municipal solid waste is recyclable. (Nearly 50 percent of all solid waste is packaging, and another 30 percent is food and yard waste.)

Recycling is certainly the most cost-effective method of dealing with the garbage crisis. Building an incinerator can cost over $500 million; a recycling program costs $5–10 million, depending on the size of the community. A study conducted in East Hampton, New York, by environmental scientist Dr. Barry Commoner of the Center for the Biology of Natural Systems at Queens College of the City University of New York, found that the cost of incinerating a ton of garbage is \$195–209, whereas the cost of recycling the same amount is \$127.

In addition to preventing the spread of toxic, cancer- causing agents into the air and into our water supplies, some additional good reasons to recycle are provided by the New York Department of Sanitation:

- A ton of recycled newsprint saves seventeen trees and can be recycled five to eight times.
- It takes an entire forest (over 500,000 trees) to supply Americans with newspapers each Sunday.
- For every job created by harvesting trees, five jobs are created by recycling the paper manufactured from those trees.
- Paper produced through recycling reduces air pollution by 20 percent and water pollution by 50 percent, and uses 30–50 percent less energy.
- Americans throw away enough office and writing paper each year to build a wall that is 7 feet high and 8½ inches wide from Los Angeles to New York.
- Americans throw out 2.5 million plastic bottles every hour; when glass containers are included, the total amount is enough to fill up the 1,350 foot tall World Trade Center Towers every two weeks.
- The United States imports 91 percent of its aluminum and throws away 1 million tons of it every year (a loss of over \$400 million).
- The energy saved by recycling one aluminum can will operate a television for three hours.
- Recycling aluminum saves up to 95 percent of the energy required to produce aluminum from ore; it also reduces air pollution by 95 percent and water pollution by 97 percent.
- Glass produced through recycling reduces air pollution by 20 percent and water pollution by 50 percent.
- Manufacturing disposable bottles requires three times as much energy as manufacturing recyclable containers.

- Discarded aluminum cans will litter the earth for 500 years, discarded glass for 1,000 years, and discarded plastic forever.

## WHAT YOU CAN DO ON A PERSONAL LEVEL

A little effort is all it takes to do your part to help save the Earth. Do not count yourself as part of a throwaway society. A few simple lifestyle changes can make a big difference.

☐ Buy less, and do not buy disposable products such as diapers, razors, and pens. Whenever possible, buy used items, such as china, flatware, books, furniture, appliances, and automobiles. Use cloth napkins and towels instead of paper, and paper garbage bags instead of plastic ones.

☐ Compost food and yard wastes (see inset on page 100). Inoculants; composting bins, tools, and other supplies; and instructions for composting are found at many nurseries and garden centers. Composting supplies are also available from the following companies:

Dirt Cheap Organics
5645 Pasadena Drive
Corte Madera, CA 94925
(415) 924-0369

Nichols Garden Nursery
1190 North Pacific Highway
Albany, OR 97321
(503) 928-9280

Gardens Alive!
PO Box 149
Sunman, IN 47041
(812) 537-8650

Peaceful Valley Farm
PO Box 2209
Grass Valley, CA 95945
(916) 272-4769

Harmonius Technology
26 North Mentor Avenue
Pasadena, CA 91106
(818) 792-2798

Seventh Generation
55 Hercules Drive
Colchester, VT 05446
(800) 456-1177

# Making a Compost Pile

*Food and yard waste account for 30 percent of all garbage. Composting is nature's perfect way of recycling this waste, while improving soil fertility.*

*To make a compost pile, you will need to clear a small area in your yard. Fill a large barrel or compost bin with a six-inch layer of dried leaves and twigs, covered with an inch of soil.*

*Add kitchen and yard wastes to the pile (but no animal meat, skin, or bones, which attract flies and foraging animals). Spray the pile with an organic inoculant to speed the composting process. Every two or three weeks, aerate the pile with a shovel or pitchfork to allow oxygen to interact with the compost ingredients. If steam rises when the pile is turned, the composting process is working efficiently.*

*Compost needs to be damp but not soggy, and if it begins to smell, it is probably too wet. Sprinkle the pile with powdered limestone (available at nurseries and garden-supply stores) and cover it with a tarpaulin. (It's a good idea to sprinkle limestone on the compost pile regularly to prevent unpleasant odors.) In dry weather, water the compost pile. With regular turning, within six to nine weeks you will have rich, dark organic matter to add to your soil.*

☐ Carry a cloth, string, or straw bag for your shopping trips. Tell the cashier you do not need a paper bag, or save the supermarket's brown shopping bags for re-use on your next trip.

☐ Return wire hangers to the dry cleaner.

☐ Re-use aluminum foil, plastic containers, and plastic food bags. Be aware: if there is any type of printing on plastic bags, do not turn the bags inside out if re-using them for food items. The printing ink on the bags may contain lead, which can leach into the food.

☐ Instead of putting unwanted clothing, furniture, and toys in the trash, see if they can be re-used. Donate them to community-service organizations such as Good-Will Industries, the Rescue Mission, the Salvation Army, and the Vietnam Veterans of America.

☐ Cut down on the amount of junk mail you receive. Have your name removed from mass-mailing lists. Send your name and address along with your request to the following address (requests must be submitted in writing).

Mail Preference Service
Direct Marketing Association
PO Box 3861
11 West 42nd Street
New York, NY 10163

☐ Air conditioners and refrigerators that were manufactured before the early 1980s may contain PCBs (polychlorinated biphenyls). These toxic chemicals are encased in metal, and normal handling is safe, but compacting or shredding them is not. Have your municipality or independent hauler cart these appliances to a toxic-waste site.

☐ Do not buy items in plastic containers that cannot be recycled in your community. (See inset on page 102.) Most plastics are not biodegradable, which means that they will remain in landfills for centuries.

☐ Call your local recycling center to find out what plastics they accept. At present, most recycling centers accept only 1/PETE and 2/HDPE, the types of plastic usually used in milk, water, juice, and soda jugs and bottles.
In an EPA ranking of the twenty chemicals whose production causes the most hazardous waste, five of the top six chemicals listed are those used in the manufacturing of plastics: propylene, phenol, ethylene, styrene, and benzene.

# Recognizing Recyclable Plastics

*In an effort to assist recycling programs, the Society of the Plastics Industry has developed a voluntary coding system (using a three-sided triangular arrow with a number from 1 to 7 in the center, and code letters beneath the number) to identify the resin composition of plastic containers. Coding symbols imprinted on the bottom of plastic containers indicate the following product composition:*

   Polyethylene Terephthalate

   High Density Polyethylene

   Vinyl/Polyvinyl Chloride

   Low Density Polyethylene

   Polypropylene

   Polystyrene

   Other Resins and Layered
Multi- Material

☐ Always cut apart the plastic rings that cover six-packs of soda and beer. Over a million sea birds and 100,000 marine animals die each year after swallowing or becoming entangled in plastic debris.

☐ Fifty percent of the mercury and cadmium in landfills comes from batteries. Discarded batteries are the cause of the most common toxic ingredients in most landfills. Buy solar-rechargeable batteries or order Varta batteries, which are mercury-free and cadmium-free, from the following companies:

Real Goods
966 Mazzoni Streeet
Ukiah, CA 95482
(800) 762-7325
*Solar-rechargable batteries*

Edward & Sons Trading Co.
Box 1326
Carpenteria, CA 93024
(805) 684-8500
*Varta batteries*

☐ Buy items with little or no packaging.

☐ Polystyrene foam, with other insulating plastics, is destroying the ozone layer. If you receive a package packed with polystyrene foam, take the foam pieces to a local packaging or shipping company for re-use. Mail Boxes, Etc., a nationwide shipping franchise with over 1,500 locations, accepts and re-uses foam pieces. Call (800) 828-2214 for the location nearest you.

☐ When you mail packages, protect the contents with crushed newspapers or popcorn, not polystyrene foam chips. In addition, use recycled and recyclable packaging materials (cushioning, mailing bags, wrapping paper, boxes, sealing tape). The following companies sell these packaging items:

American Excelsior Co.
PO Box 5067
Arlington, TX 76005
(817) 640-1555

Eco-Pack Industries, Inc.
20648 84th Avenue South
Kent, WA 98032
(206) 251-0918

☐ Recycle all paper, glass, metal, and aluminum. If you have items that your local recycling program does not pick up, call your municipality or the League of Women Voters to find out where to take the recyclables.

☐ Some gas stations accept used motor oil for recycling. Find out which gas stations in your neighborhood offer this service.

☐ Buy recycled paper products. It is important for us, as consumers, to support the need for all kinds of recycled paper products. Many grocery stores and natural foods stores carry these items. Recycled paper products are also available from the following companies:

Atlantic Recycled Paper
PO Box 39096
Baltimore, MD 21212
(800) 323-2811
*Full line of home and office supplies.*

Bandelier Designs
PO Box 9656
Santa Fe, NM 87504
(505) 986-1600
*Full line of stationery and stationery accessories.*

Conservatree Paper
Suite 250
10 Lombard Street
San Francisco, CA 94111
(800) 522-9200
*Full line of office supplies and stationery.*

Earth Care Paper
PO Box 7070
Madison, WI 53707
(608) 277-2900
*Full line of office supplies and stationery.*

EcoLogicals
1167 Route 52 – Suite 226
Fishkill, NY 12524
(914) 897-3411
*Full line of home and office supplies.*

Seventh Generation
55 Hercules Drive
Colchester, VT 05446
(800) 456-1177
*Full line of household products.*

☐ Use natural household cleaners and cosmetics (see Chapters 16 and 28). If you do, however, use commercial products, do not dispose of the empty containers in your household garbage. Take them to a hazardous-waste site. Other containers to be disposed of in hazardous-waste sites include those that held automotive supplies (anti-freeze, transmission fluid, motor oil, fuel, polish, and wax); photographic and paint supplies; wood-working supplies (glue, cement, and preservatives); garden supplies (herbicides, insecticides, and weed killers); mothballs; metal polishes; solvents (rust remover and turpentine); flammable fuels; nail polish remover; and any other chemicals. Call your municipality to find out when a hazardous-waste collection is planned.

☐ Never bury toxic materials along the side of a road or pour toxic-waste products down a storm drain or street sewer. Read all labels on toxic materials carefully. Observe the precautions for use and follow the recommendations for disposal.

☐ Raise your consciousness. Use less, and there will be less to dispose of. At present, with 6 percent of the world's population, the United States uses 60 percent of the world's resources.

☐ The following companies sell a wide range of natural, biodegradable, and recycled products. Write or call for a free catalogue.

Co-op America
Suite 403
2100 M Street, NW
Washington, DC 20036
(202) 223-1881

Earth Products
3441 South Lincoln Drive
Englewood, CO 80110
(800) 875-0224

The Ecology Box
2260 South Main Street
Ann Arbor, MI 48103
(800) 735-1371
(313) 662-9131

EcoSource Products
380-F Morris Street
Sebastopol, CA 95472
(707) 829-7562

Karen's Nontoxic Products
1839 Dr. Jack Road
Conowingo, MD 21918
(800) KARENS-4

NEEDS
527 Charles Avenue
Syracuse, NY 13209
(800) 634-1380

Non-Polluting Enterprises
  (NOPE)
Suite 5E
342 West 21st Street
New York, NY 10011
(800) 782-NOPE
(212) 989-4222

Real Goods
966 Mazzoni Street
Ukiah, CA 95482
(800) 762-7325

Seventh Generation
55 Hercules Drive
Colchester, VT 05446
(800) 456-1177

☐ *101 Practical Tips for Home and Work: Recycling* by Susan Hassol and Beth Richman is an informative book on recycling. For a copy of this work, send your request along with a check or money order in the amount of $5.00 (price includes shipping and handling) to:

The Windstar Foundation
2317 Snowmass Creek Road
Snowmass, CO 81654
(303) 927-4777

**HOW TO GET MORE INVOLVED**

Show your concern on matters dealing with garbage reduction and recycling. In addition to following the suggestions in the previous section of this chapter, there are other things you can do.

☐ If recycling is not already an integral part of your municipal service, urge your local legislators to implement a program.

☐ Write to manufacturers and urge them to reduce the amount of packaging that is used for their products, especially if bubble wrap or polystyrene foam (chips or peanuts) is used.

☐ Raise your consciousness. Look for further information, including updated reports on issues of landfill disposal and incineration hazards, recycling tips, and methods to reduce garbage volume. Contact the following organizations for up-to-date information. (Additional information on the organizations is found beginning on page 269.)

Clean Water Action
1320 18th Street, NW
Washington, DC 20036
(202) 457-1286

Citizens Clearinghouse
  for Hazardous Waste
PO Box 6806
Falls Church, VA 22040

Friends of the Earth
215 D Street, SE
Washington, DC 20003
(202) 544-2600

Greenpeace International
1436 U Street, NW
Washington, DC 20077
(202) 462-1177

INFORM, Inc.
381 Park Avenue South
New York, NY 10016
(212) 689-4040

U.S. Public Interest
  Research Group
215 Pennsylvania Avenue, SE
Washington, DC 20003
(202) 546-9707

# Chapter 15

# HAZARDOUS-WASTE SITES

Hazardous waste is discarded material of a chemical nature that, if disposed of improperly, could pose a threat to human health, life, and to the environment. The EPA estimates that in the United States approximately 534 million tons of hazardous waste are generated annually (more than two tons per person).

Most hazardous waste is produced by industry, and over 90 percent of it is stored on the sites where it is generated. Hazardous waste is usually disposed of either by dumping in landfills, pits, ponds, or lagoons; by incineration; or through the process known as *land farming*. In the land-farming process, wastes are mixed with surface soil, and the microbial action in the soil hastens the degradation process.

Hazardous waste includes heavy metals such as arsenic, cadmium, chromium, and lead; organics such as PCBs (polychlorinated biphenyls), fungicides, herbicides, rodenticides, esters, ethers, chlorinated hydrocarbons, dioxins, and various amides, amines, and imides (the basic building blocks in chemical and plastics production); trichloroethylene (TCE); benzene; and asbestos. All of these chemicals can cause cancer. Hazardous waste also includes components that can cause birth defects and genetic damage, and/or materials such as manganese and mercury, which can damage the brain, central nervous system, respiratory system, and digestive system.

The first federal program to clean up uncontrolled hazardous-waste sites was created in 1980 by the federal Comprehensive Environmental Response Compensation and Liability Act (CERCLA). CERCLA was amended in 1986 under the Superfund Amendments and Reauthorization Act (SARA), which was signed into law just as our national consciousness was being raised by the 1978 Hooker Chemical (now renamed Occidental Petroleum) disaster at Love Canal. In 1978, residents of the neighborhood next to Love Canal, several miles outside the town of Niagara Falls, New York, became alarmed as sticky black sludge oozed into their basements, acrid fumes from heat vents filled their living rooms, and puddles of caustic, pastel-colored water formed on their lawns. State technicians tested the air in the home of Aileen and Edwin Voorhees, and found elevated levels of seven chemicals. These chemicals posed a health risk that was 5,000 times higher than normal.

It was discovered that the source of these toxic components was the Love Canal, an abandoned hydroelectric channel into which Hooker Chemical had dumped 44 million pounds of toxic sludge, solvents, and pesticide residues—including the potent carcinogens benzene and dioxin—since 1948. The chemicals were eventually carried throughout the neighborhood via surrounding sewers and creeks.

Beverly Paigen, a researcher at Roswell Park Memorial Institute in Buffalo, New York, found evidence that residents of the area had increased risks of miscarriage, low birth weight, and birth defects; and that children who lived close to the canal suffered from learning disabilities, seizures, hyperactivity, skin and eye irritation, and urinary incontinence.

The evacuation of 1,004 families from the Love Canal area took place between 1978 and 1980. Houses that were adjacent to the canal were bulldozed under. The canal is now capped with clay and surrounded by a drainage system that intercepts any sludge that migrates from the site. Nearby creeks have been fenced off to keep children away. The Department of Health and Human Services began to form a registry of the estimated 5,000 to 10,000 people who lived near the Love Canal from 1948 to 1978. It is difficult to conduct a conclusive study, however, because of the limited population, the multiple health disorders, the unknown effects of chemicals when they interact, and the fact that it is difficult to track residents who move in and out.

Following the incident at Love Canal, $1.6 billion was appropriated and a nationwide five-year cleanup of hazardous waste sites began. At the end of five years, however, only a handful of sites had been treated. At several of these sites, costly remedies had failed on a spectacular scale.

In some cases, wastes that were left on site were not properly contained. In other cases, hazardous waste was moved from original sites to new sites. The new sites became contaminated so quickly that they were soon added to the list of Superfund dumps. Groups of citizens who were most affected by the proximity of designated sites were excluded from the EPA's decision-making process on cleanup planning. Industries that had polluted the sites were themselves put in charge of cleaning them up. EPA standards for "safe" levels of toxic and carcinogenic chemicals varied widely from site to site.

In 1983, the EPA designated the Lipari Landfill, in Pitman, New Jersey—a former sand and gravel pit—as the nation's number one cleanup priority. The Lipari Landfill is a few hundred feet from a residential neighborhood and just upshore from placid Lake Alcyon. Today, signs continue to warn residents and visitors not to fish, swim, water ski, or boat there. Over a thirteen-year period, three million gallons of chemical waste had been legally deposited at the fifteen-acre Lipari Landfill by approximately sixty companies. Among the companies dumping the greatest volume of waste were Rohm and Haas, Owens-Illinois, Inc., and CBS Records.

By 1971, the residents of Pitman and the neighboring towns of Harrison and Glassboro had complained of respiratory problems, nausea, dying vegetation, and noxious odors and fumes that regularly brought tears to their eyes, so the landfill was closed. Reports of health problems continued, however, and the once-pristine waters of Lake Alcyon continued to turn orange and purple. In 1979, tests showed that among other toxic chemicals leaking into the lake there were trace levels of the carcinogens bis (2-chlorethyl) ether, methylene chloride, and benzene.

To demonstrate serious intent and effective policy, the government decided to clean up Lipari as a demonstration project, and spent $750,000 and several years studying the problem. In 1983, the EPA announced a $2.1 million containment plan: an underground wall would isolate and contain the chemicals, preventing further seepage, and a protective polyethylene cap would cover the site. The wall and cap were completed within a year, but foul, chemical odors continued to sicken area residents. Each day, some 2,600 gallons of waste continued to leak through the wall and through the fractured, natural clay substrata beneath the landfill. (Prior to 1983, over 100,000 gallons had leaked from the site every day.)

In 1985, against the advice of state investigators and its own consultants, the EPA began a seven-year flushing of the landfill's chemicals and initiated an on-site treatment program. The treatment plant was completed in 1991. It is expected that by the year 2000, the contaminants in the site's toxic sludge will be reduced significantly, so that they will no longer pose a threat to the environment or the community's health. The estimated cost of the flush-and-treatment program for the Lipari Landfill and of the cleaning up of Lake Alcyon is over $40 million.

Meanwhile, the New Jersey State Department of Health found in 1989 that people living within 1 kilometer (five-eighths of a mile) of the Lipari Landfill were at risk of developing adult leukemia and of producing children with low birth weight. The Department continues to monitor and register low birth weight and cancer cases among current and former Pitman residents.

The Superfund has been plagued by reported instances of inefficiency and fraud. In 1983, former program director Rita Lavelle was convicted of lying in order to cover up a toxic-dump investigation. To date, the EPA has suspended contracts with seven labs. At least ten other labs have been and continue to be investigated for alleged fraud in reporting false chemical test results. Environmental activists fear that polluters, who now must foot most of the cleanup bills, may plea bargain, striking deals with the EPA that will provide only temporary solutions.

By all estimates, the cleanup will be a Herculean task that could take decades. Nearly 2,000 hazardous-waste sites are scheduled for cleanup by the end of 1992. Additionally, the Pentagon says it knows of 11,000 contaminated sites at military bases nationwide. (On the EPA's list of 116 most dangerous sites, 95 are military bases.) Between 1979 and 1991, approximately 40 sites had been cleaned up and removed from the official list. The true number of sites may be much higher because new sites are being identified all the time, and some sites that have been closed or abandoned have not yet been examined. On some of these closed and abandoned sites, schools, offices, and houses have been built, and community activities are taking place. As of 1991, estimates for cleanup at each site averaged $26 million—half of it for legal and administrative fees. The Congressional Office of Technology Assessment estimates that the total cleanup cost could exceed $500 billion over the next 50 years, and other estimates have run as high as $1 trillion, including $200 billion in transaction costs (mostly legal fees).

The only available solutions to a problem site are monitoring, neutralization, destruction, encapsulation, or removal of the waste to a safer site. Most treatments of hazardous waste are not remedies at all; they merely minimize the damage to the environment and the threats to local residents' health, including the risk of cancer. Even when these threats are diluted, clusters of cancer may continue to occur in communities where hazardous waste has been dumped.

## WHAT YOU CAN DO ON A PERSONAL LEVEL

Protect yourself against the hazards resulting from toxic-waste sites. The following suggestions will prove helpful.

☐ Before buying a new home, contact the EPA and your community environmental-action organizations for information. Have them confirm that there is no toxic-waste site near the property you have chosen.

☐ Citizens Clearinghouse for Hazardous Waste publishes a thorough and informative guide called *Environmental Testing*. Its step-by-step program is designed to determine whether a problem exists, how widespread it is, how to evaluate potential health problems, and how to gather exposure data. For a copy of this publication, send your request along with a check or money order in the amount of $12.04 (price includes shipping and handling) to:

> Citizens Clearinghouse
>    for Hazardous Waste
> PO Box 6806
> Falls Church, VA 22040

☐ The EPA has flagged the following industries as the largest producers of hazardous waste. Go to your local library and check the *Thomas Register of American Manufacturers* and *Dalton's Directory* to see whether manufacturers in these industries are located in your neighborhood or community. Your chamber of commerce can also supply this information.

Manufacturers of:

| | |
|---|---|
| Batteries | Paint and allied products |
| Electronic components | Pesticides |
| Explosives | Pharmaceuticals |
| Ferrous metals | Plastics and synthetics |
| Inorganic chemicals | Special machinery |
| Non-ferrous metals | Textile-mill products |
| Organic chemicals | |

Also, industries for:

Electroplating
Leather tanning
Petroleum refining

☐  For a free copy of the report *Superfund: Focusing on the Nation at Large*, which includes the most dangerous hazardous-waste sites on the National Priorities List, and for more detailed information on your state's sites, write to:

EPA
ORD Publications, Room G-72
26 West Martin Luther King Drive
Cincinnati, OH 45268
(513) 569-7562
(When ordering, ask for EPA document number 540/8-90/009.)

The EPA also has Superfund Community Specialists at each regional office. To locate your nearest EPA center, call (800) 424-9346, or look for the EPA Public Affairs Office in the white pages of your telephone book.

## HOW TO GET MORE INVOLVED

The following suggestions are offered to better protect you against dangers from toxic waste.

☐  If you know of or think there is a toxic-waste dump in your community, contact the Sierra Club, Environmental Action Foundation, and the Citizens Clearinghouse for Hazardous Waste (addresses on page 116). These groups have successful track records as environmental problem-solvers, and their network of environmental activists can help identify the scope of the problem, focus community attention on it, and help find a solution.

The Sierra Club and the Environmental Action Foundation publish guidelines for a "Hunt the Dump Campaign," a strategy that evaluates manufacturing companies' disposal sites and teaches how to stimulate public and governmental awareness of potential hazards.

☐  Commit yourself to further involvement by supporting the following organizations, which either disseminate pertinent information on hazardous waste or lobby for stricter controls and cleanup campaigns. (Additional information on the organizations is found beginning on page 269.)

Citizens Clearinghouse
  for Hazardous Waste
PO Box 6806
Falls Church, VA 22040
(703) 237-CCHW

Clean Water Action
Suite 300
1320 18th Street, NW
Washington, DC 20036
(202) 457-1286

Environmental Action
6930 Carroll Avenue
Tacoma Park, MD 20912
(301) 891-1100

Environmental Defense Fund
257 Park Avenue South
New York, NY 10010
(212) 505-2100

Friends of the Earth
218 D Street, SE
Washington, DC 20003
(202) 544-2600

Greenpeace International
1436 U Street, NW
Washington, DC 20077
(202) 462-1177

INFORM, Inc.
381 Park Avenue South
New York, NY 10016
(212) 689-4040

Sierra Club
730 Polk Street
San Francisco, CA 94109
(415) 923-5653

# Chapter 16

# INDOOR POLLUTION AND HOUSEHOLD PRODUCTS

There are approximately 4 million chemical compounds present in our environment. Some 63,000 chemicals are found in homes throughout the United States in such common products as clothing, sheets, towels, carpeting, kitchen counters and cabinets, cosmetics, paints, adhesives, paper towels, and grocery bags. An estimated one thousand new chemicals are synthesized every day. Many of these chemicals are toxic, and as they interact with other compounds in the environment, their harmful effects can be multiplied.

The National Academy of Sciences Board on Environmental Studies and Toxicology estimates that 15 percent of the population is hypersensitive to chemicals present in common household products; some people are physically intolerant of even very small amounts. Pollution from an individual source may not be a risk in itself, but most homes have many sources, and the cumulative exposure can result in serious health problems.

Many chemicals in household products cause cancer. Additionally, they may cause headaches; intestinal cramps; nausea; irritation of the eyes, nose, and sinus cavities; blurred vision; mental confusion; incoherent speech; memory loss; fatigue; tension; depression; joint and muscle pain and spasms; eczema and other skin rashes; and a host of other ailments.

From 1980 to 1985, an EPA Total Exposure Assessment Methodology (TEAM) study confirmed that measurements of indoor toxic chemical levels are significantly higher than outdoor levels, even in the largest and most industrialized cities; and most people spend 90 percent of their time indoors. People most exposed to indoor pollutants generally include those who might be the most susceptible to their harmful effects: the young, the old, and the chronically ill.

Table 16.1 lists common household products and building materials that contribute to indoor pollution, together with their harmful ingredients (many are known or suspected carcinogens). Also provided is a list of recommended alternatives. Not every product on the market necessarily contains the chemicals or contaminants specified in Table 16.1. To be sure of the contents of a particular product, you must either read the label or contact the manufacturer. Most recommended alternative products listed in Table 16.1 are available in hardware stores, supermarkets, and natural foods stores. In addition, the mail-order companies listed in Table 16.1 also sell the recommended products (addresses found beginning on page 126).

**Table 16.1  Safe Alternatives for Common Household Products and Materials**

| Product | Problem | Solution |
|---|---|---|
| Adhesives, glues | May contain naphthalene, phenol, ethanol, vinyl chloride, formaldehyde, andacrylonitrile. | Use white glue and carpenter's glue, which are safe when dry. Use natural, nontoxic adhesive products available in many hardware stores, and from AFM Enterprises, EcoDesign Company, Master's Corporation, and Karen's Nontoxic Products. |
| Aerosols | Contain PVP (polyvinyl pyrrolidinone) and CFCs (chlorofluorocarbons). | Select products in pump sprays. |

| Product | Problem | Solution |
|---|---|---|
| Air fresheners | May contain petroleum distillates (benzene, trichloroethylene, perchloroethylene, PDB [paradichlorobenzene]), cresol, formaldehyde, phenol, napthalene, xylene, and ethanol. | Freshen the air with bowls of baking soda or mixtures of baking soda and water, herbal mixtures, or potpourri. |
| All-purpose cleaners | Many contain ammonia, petroleum distillates, PDB (paradichlorobenzene), and chlorine. | Make your own all-purpose cleaner by combining 1 gallon warm water, ¼ cup white vinegar, and 1 teaspoon baking soda. Purchase nontoxic cleaners found in hardware stores and natural foods stores, or from Earth Rite, NEEDS, Seventh Generation, Shaklee, The Allergy Store, The Ecology Box, The Living Source, Nontoxic Environments, Karen's Nontoxic Products, and Granny's Old-Fashioned Products. |
| Carpet and rug cleaners | Most contain perchloroethylene, trichloroethylene, ethanol. | To keep carpets fresh, sprinkle with baking soda or borax, then vacuum. To remove stains, wash carpeting with mild soapy water and rinse with a mixture of 3 parts water and 1 part vinegar. |
| Carpets, rugs, backings | Often contain a host of chemicals used as stain repellents, biocides, and fungicides. | Consider natural wood, tile, or a polished concrete floor. Handmade area rugs are usually toxin free. Nylon is the most benign synthetic material. Use jute, not polyurethane, as backing. AFM Enterprises sells safe carpet sealers. |

| Product | Problem | Solution |
|---------|---------|----------|
| Caulking compounds | Many contain xylene, phenol, asbestos. | Use Dap Kwik Seal Tub & Tile Caulk. Other nontoxic caulking compounds are found in most hardware stores or from AFM Enterprises and Nontoxic Environments. |
| Charcoal lighters | Contain napthalene. | Use paper or kindling. |
| Countertops | Plastic laminate materials, such as Formica, are usually applied over a particleboard core, which gives off formaldehyde fumes. | When ordering countertops, make sure laminate is applied to exterior-grade plywood and is sealed on both sides. Consider countertops made of tile or Corian (a solid material made by DuPont), which is seemingly benign to the homeowner. |
| Dish and laundry detergents | Most contain surfactants; dodecylbenzol derivatives; polyoxy alkalene; sorbitan alkylates, mono-laureates, and mono-oleates. | Try equal parts borax and water. Natural, environmentally safe dish and laundry soaps can be purchased at most natural foods stores, or from Shaklee, Granny's Old-Fashioned Products, Living Source, Seventh Generation, NEEDS, NOPE, The Ecology Box, Nontoxic Environments. |
| Disinfectants | Often contain ammonia, cresol, phenolethanol, formaldehyde. | Use a mixture of ½ cup borax and 1 gallon hot water. |
| Drain cleaners | Most contain lye, hydrochloric acid, sulfuric acid, and phosphoric acid. | Use a plunger or snake for blockages. For preventive maintenance, each week pour a mixture of ½ cup washing soda dissolved in 1 quart of hot water down drains. |

| Product | Problem | Solution |
|---|---|---|
| Drapes, upholstery fabrics | Often contain formaldehyde, plasticizers, dye residues, fungicides. | Use untreated, natural materials such as cotton, wool, linen, horsehair, and down. |
| Dry cleaning sprays and fluids | Contain benzene, toluene, perchloroethylene, trichloroethylene, tetrachloroethylene. | Wash clothing in cold water and pure soap. Nontoxic stain removers can be purchased from Granny's Old-Fashioned Products. |
| Dyes | Many contain coal tar by-products, benzene, toluene, naphthalene, phenol, cresol, dichlorobenzene. | Use vegetable dyes, natural dyes, and colorfast dyes that are not released by perspiration and absorbed into the skin. |
| Fabric softeners | Contain surfactants. | In final rinse of the wash cycle add ¼ cup baking soda. |
| Furniture | Often made of particleboard or other wood products that contain formaldehyde. | When possible, choose furniture made of solid wood, metal, or natural materials (bamboo, wicker, etc.). If furniture is constructed of particleboard, be sure to seal any exposed areas. (See Particleboard.) |
| Furniture polish and floor wax (for wood) | Most contain nitrobenzene, phenol, ammonia, petroleum distillates. | Use microcrystalline paste wax. Nontoxic wood polishes are found in some hardware stores or can be purchased from Bau/Biofa, Eco Design Company, Nontoxic Environments, and Sinan. |
| Glass cleaners | May include naphthalene, ammonia. | Make your own glass-cleaning solutions. Use mixture of ¼ cup of white vinegar and 1 quart of warm water, or add 2 tablespoons of borax and 2 tablespoons of washing soda to 3 cups of water. Nontoxic glass cleaners are found in some supermarkets and most natural foods stores. |

| Product | Problem | Solution |
| --- | --- | --- |
| Insecticides | Contain a wide variety of toxic chemicals. | See Chapter 20 for nontoxic alternatives to get rid of bugs. |
| Insulation materials (fiberglass batts, rigid foam panels, blown-in cellulose) | Fiberglass contains glass fibers, which, when inhaled, can lodge in respiratory tract; can also irritate eyes and skin. Cellulose and rigid foam panels contain various chemical compounds. | Use particle-filter dust mask during handling and installation of fiberglass or cellulose insulation. Ventilate house well after installation. Make sure no insulation is exposed. Natural cork is an expensive option. Another less expensive option is Air-Krete, a nontoxic, magnesium oxide-based foam available from Master's Corporation. |
| Metal polishes | Most contain ammonia, lye, hydrochloric acid, sulfuric acid, and phosphoric acid. | Make your own nontoxic polish by mixing calcium carbonate (whiting) with olive oil to make a paste. |
| Mold and mildew cleaners | Many contain formaldehyde, phenol, pentachlorophenol, DDVP (dimethyldichlorovinylphosphate), PDB (paradichlorobenzene), kerosene. | Use borax. Many hardware stores and most natural foods stores carry nontoxic mold and mildew cleaners. Products are also available from AFM Enterprises, NEEDS, The Allergy Store, Nontoxic Environments, and The Ecology Box. |
| Mothballs | Contain DDVP (dimethyldichlorovinyl phosphate), PDB (paradichlorobenzene). | Use cedar chips, lavender sachets, and herbal sachets. |
| Oven cleaners | Some contain surfactants, lye, hydrochloric acid, sulfuric acid, and phosphoric acid. | Set a bowl of ammonia in the oven overnight. In the morning, wipe the oven clean. |

| Product | Problem | Solution |
|---|---|---|
| Paints (oil-based, acrylic, alkyd) | Contain toxic hydrocarbon solvents; may contain chromium, cobalt, cadmium, formaldehyde, PCBs (polychlorinated biphenyls), fungicides, benzene, kerosene, methylene chloride, lead. | Use whitewash or casein-based milk paints. Low or nontoxic paint products are sold in some hardware stores and can be ordered from AFM Enterprises, Eco Design, EcoSource, The Ecology Box, and Nontoxic Environments. |
| Particleboard (used for floor underlayment; roof and wall sheathing; shelving; core stock for plastic laminate countertops, cupboards, and bathroom vanities; furniture framing; interior doors; stair treads; television and stereo housings) | Contains urea-formaldehyde, reportedly up to 10 percent by weight, which can give off fumes for years after manufacture. | Use pine boards or other solid woods whenever possible. Seal exposed (not necessarily visible) surfaces of existing particleboard products—such as bottom faces of laminate counters and inside surfaces and edges of cupboards and vanities. Latex paint won't seal in vapors; use two coats of alkyd-base paint and ventilate area until dry. |
| Pens and markers (permanent ink) | Contain acetone, cresol, ethanol, phenol, toluene, xylene. | Use water-based markers and pens. |
| Plywood, hardwood (interior paneling, furniture, cabinetry veneers) | Contains urea-formaldehyde resins, although in lower concentrations than in particleboard. | Use solid pine paneling. If hardwood plywood is used, seal all surfaces as with particleboard. |
| Plywood, softwood—meaning all common structural grades (subflooring; wall and roof sheathing; some furniture, cabinets, and shelving) | Interior grades contain urea-formaldehyde resins. Exterior grades (water resistant) contain phenol-formaldehyde resins, which are likely to produce less of the noxious fumes. | If you must use plywood, use exterior grades. Seal all surfaces as with particleboard. |

| Product | Problem | Solution |
|---|---|---|
| Scouring powder | May contain talc, chlorine. | Use a paste made of baking soda and water. |
| Shoe polish | Most contain a host of hazardous chemicals including nitrobenzene, perchloroethylene, trichloroethylene, coal-tar dyes. | Use nut oils as a nontoxic substitute for shoe polish. Other chemical-free shoe products are available from AFM Enterprises, Eco Design Company, and Nontoxic Environments. |
| Soaps (body) | Often contain phenol, petroleum distillates, BHA (butylated hydroxyanisole), BHT (butylated hydroxytoluene), formaldehyde, ammonia. | Use pure, unscented soap. Most natural foods stores carry pure body soaps. |
| Soaps (laundry). *See* Dish and Laundry Soaps. | | |
| Spot removers | Most contain trichloroethylene, perchloroethylene. | Make your own spot remover by combining ¼ cup of borax and 2 cups of cold water. Nontoxic spot remover is available from Granny's Old-Fashioned Products. |
| Toilet bowl cleaners | Contain formaldehyde, surfactants, chloride, lye, hydrochloric acid, sulfuric acid, and phosphoric acid. | Use borax or a mixture of 1 cup hydrogen peroxide and 2 quarts water. Let stand in toilet bowl 30 minutes, brush, and flush. For stains, use a paste mixture of borax and lemon juice. |
| Turpentine | Includes toluene, xylene. | Use nontoxic mineral spirits. |
| Typewriter correction fluid | Contains cresol, ethanol, napthalene, trichloroethylene. | Use white-out tape or typewriter ink erasers. |

| Product | Problem | Solution |
|---|---|---|
| Varnishes and sealants | Most contain toxic hydrocarbon solvents, phenol, and petroleum distillates. | Use shellac. |
| Vinyl floor coverings | Contain plasticizers. | If vinyl tiles are used, select hard tiles rather than soft ones. Hard vinyl contains less plasticizers. |
| Wall coverings | Vinyl wall coverings may have outgassing from plasticizers. Wallpaper adhesive may contain fungicides and mildewcides. | Choose paper, linen, or foil wall coverings. Use low-toxic adhesives, which are available from AFM Enterprises and Master's Corporation. |
| Wood finishes and preservatives | May contain mildewcides, fungicides, and a variety of toxic solvents. May include benzene, lead, formaldehyde, acronylitrile, creosote, and pentachlorophenol. | Use water- or casein-based products. Products are found in many hardware stores or can be ordered from Eco Design, Nontoxic Environments, and Karen's Nontoxic Products. If possible, use naturally rot-resistant woods (redwood, cedar). |

Some of the information presented in this table has been adapted (with permission) from the article "Sick Home Blues" by Peter Fossel, as it appeared in the September/October 1987 issue of *Harrowsmith Country Life*, Ferry Road, Charlotte, VT 05445.

## WHAT YOU CAN DO ON A PERSONAL LEVEL

A few lifestyle changes can make a healthy difference in the indoor air quality of your home.

☐ Keep your house well ventilated. An air-tight home with extra insulation, caulking, and weatherstripping does not provide a healthy environment. If too little outdoor air enters a home, pollutants can accumulate at levels that cause discomfort and illness. If your home was built to be energy-efficient and is tightly weatherproofed, you can increase ventilation mechanically with a heat-recovery ventilator, also known as an air-to-air heat exchanger. This two-way ventilator draws outdoor air into the house and recovers the heat from the indoor air before exhausting it to the outside.

An air-to-air heat exchanger system that also removes gases, dust, and pollens, and maintains balanced humidity levels, is available from

Berner Air Products, Inc.
PO Box 5410
New Castle, PA 16105
(800) 852-5015

☐ Use chemical-free household products (see Table 16.1). Many of the alternative products listed in the Table are available in some supermarkets, hardware stores, and most natural foods stores. Following is a list of mail-order companies that also sell nontoxic alternative products for your home. Call for a free copy of their product catalogues.

AFM Enterprises
ll40 Stacy Court
Riverside, CA 92507
(714) 781-6860
*Household cleaning products; all-natural wall paints, adhesives, sealers; carpet guard.*

Bau/Biofa
PO Box 190
Alton, NH 03809
(603) 364-2400
*All-natural wall paints, floor varnish, and household cleaning products.*

The Allergy Store
PO Box 2555
Sebastopol, CA 95473
(800) 824-7163
(707) 823-6202
*Household cleaning products.*

Co-op America
PO Box 18217
Washington, DC 20036
(800) 424-2667
*Household cleaning products; natural-fiber clothing, rugs, pillows, towels, and luggage.*

Eco Design Company
1365 Rufina Circle
Santa Fe, NM 87501
(505) 988-9111
*Household cleaning products; all-natural paints, stains, wood-finish products; glues and adhesives.*

EcoLogicals
Suite 226
1167 Route 52
Fishkill, NY 12524
(914) 897-3411
*Household cleaning products.*

The Ecology Box
Room 202
2260 South Main Street
Ann Arbor, MI 48103
(800) 735-1371
(313) 662-9131
*Household cleaning products.*

EcoSource
PO Box 1656
Sebastopol, CA 95473
(800) 274-7040
*Household cleaning products; all-natural paints, sealants, stains.*

Granny's Old-Fashioned
  Products
PO Box 256
Arcadia, CA 91066
(800) 366-1762
(818) 577-1825
*Household cleaning products; stain-removal products.*

Karen's Nontoxic Products
1839 Dr. Jack Road
Conowingo, MD 21918
(800) KARENS-4
*Household cleaning products; all-natural cleaning tools and equipment; air-therapy products; all-natural wall paints, adhesives, sealers; unbleached, undyed cotton products (diapers, towels, clothing).*

The Living Source
Suite 214
7005 Woodway Drive
Waco, TX 76712
(817) 776-4878
*Household cleaning products; nontoxic building materials.*

Masters Corporation
4 Forest Street
New Canaan, CT 06840
(203) 966-3541
*Full lines of all-natural paints, stains, sealants, adhesives; non-toxic building materials (recycled lumber, cork insulation); nontoxic wall and floor coverings.*

NEEDS
Suite 12A
527 Charles Avenue
Syracuse, NY 13209
(800) 634-1380
(315) 488-6300
*Household cleaning products; all-natural fiber clothing (T-shirts, shorts, sweatclothes); paints and adhesives; air-purification products.*

Non-Polluting Enterprises
   (NOPE)
PO Box 919D
Old Chelsea Station
New York, NY 10011
(800) 782-NOPE
(212) 727-9249
*Natural-fiber rugs, shower curtains,*
*sponges, and string bags.*

Nontoxic Environments
6135 NW Mountain View Dr.
Corvallis, OR 97330
(503) 745-7838
*Nontoxic building materials; paints,*
*sealants, finishes, and adhesives;*
*floor coverings; household cleaning*
*products; natural-fiber bedding.*

Seventh Generation
49 Hercules Drive
Colchester, VT 05446
(800) 456-1177
*Nontoxic household cleaning prod-*
*ucts; natural-fiber clothing, bedding,*
*linens.*

Shaklee
444 Market Street
San Francisco, CA 94111
(800) SHAKLEE
*Nontoxic household cleaning prod-*
*ucts.*

Sinan Company
PO Box 857
Davis, CA 95617
(916) 753-3104
*Nontoxic building materials; paints,*
*sealants, waxes, and polishes; floor*
*coverings.*

☐ If you must use a toxic product, be sure to wear a protective mask and use the product in a well-ventilated area.

☐ Buy non-aerosol products. Aerosols contain hydrocarbons, and when these compounds combine with oxides of nitrogen in the presence of sunlight, ground-level ozone (a major component of smog) is formed. Polluting compounds may be in the propellant or in the spray itself.

☐ If you use sprays (aerosol or non-aerosol), leave the area after spraying; particles in the spray can remain airborne for several minutes, and, if inhaled, can lodge in the lungs. Ozone-damaging CFCs (chlorofluorocarbons) were banned as aerosol propellants in 1978, but other toxic ingredients in propelled mist attach themselves to dust motes and remain airborne. These toxins are easily inhaled for long periods after the spray appears to have settled.

Pump-spray containers (11-ounce size) for cosmetics, degreasers, paints, air fresheners, lubricants—that use normal air instead of gas propellants—are available for under $10.00 from the following company:

LDSystems, Inc.
908 South Tryon Street – Suite 2200
Charlotte, NC 28202
(704) 332-2336

☐ Many other chemicals that are not linked specifically to cancer are associated with diseases of the heart, lungs, and central nervous system. Among the most dangerous of these chemicals are lye, hydrochloric acid, sulfuric acid, and phosphoric acid. These chemicals are found in some oven cleaners, drain cleaners, toilet cleaners, and metal polishes. Ammonia— another dangerous chemical—is found in many all-purpose cleaners, glass cleaners, disinfectants, and metal polishes. For a listing of all toxic products and their health effects, read:

*Clinical Toxicology of Consumer Products*, edited by R.E. Gosslin. Baltimore: Williams and Wilkins Co., 1984.

☐ To help keep the air in your home clean, ban smoking in your house.

☐ Air all newly dry-cleaned articles outdoors before using or wearing them. The chemicals used in dry-cleaning (benzene, toluene, perchloroethylene, trichloroethylene, and tetrachloroethylene) cause cancer in animals and may cause cancer in humans.

☐ Make sure all household appliances are vented outdoors. Household appliances are major sources of nitrogen dioxide and carbon monoxide. If your gas flame is yellow or orange, it is emitting too much carbon monoxide and needs to be adjusted.

# Making Your Own
# Nontoxic Products

*The following recipes are provided to help you reduce the indoor pollution in your home.*

### All-Purpose Cleaner

*1 gallon water*
*¼ cup white vinegar*
*1 tablespoon baking soda*

1. In a pail or basin, mix the ingredients together.
2. Use as you would a commercial all-purpose cleaner.

### Drain Cleaner

*¼ cup baking soda*
*½ cup vinegar*
*Boiling water*

1. Pour baking soda down blocked drain followed by vinegar. Close drain.
2. When fizzing stops, flush drain with boiling water.
3. For regular maintenance, flush drains with ½ cup washing soda dissolved in a quart of hot water. Do this weekly.

### Glass and Chrome Cleaner

*¼ cup white vinegar*
*1 quart warm water*

1. In a pail or basin, mix ingredients together.
2. Use as you would a commercial glass/chrome cleaner.

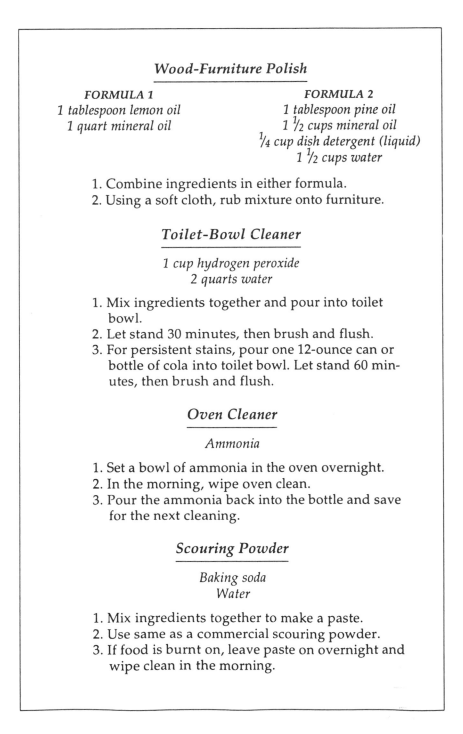

### Wood-Furniture Polish

*FORMULA 1*
*1 tablespoon lemon oil*
*1 quart mineral oil*

*FORMULA 2*
*1 tablespoon pine oil*
*1 ½ cups mineral oil*
*¼ cup dish detergent (liquid)*
*1 ½ cups water*

1. Combine ingredients in either formula.
2. Using a soft cloth, rub mixture onto furniture.

### Toilet-Bowl Cleaner

*1 cup hydrogen peroxide*
*2 quarts water*

1. Mix ingredients together and pour into toilet bowl.
2. Let stand 30 minutes, then brush and flush.
3. For persistent stains, pour one 12-ounce can or bottle of cola into toilet bowl. Let stand 60 minutes, then brush and flush.

### Oven Cleaner

*Ammonia*

1. Set a bowl of ammonia in the oven overnight.
2. In the morning, wipe oven clean.
3. Pour the ammonia back into the bottle and save for the next cleaning.

### Scouring Powder

*Baking soda*
*Water*

1. Mix ingredients together to make a paste.
2. Use same as a commercial scouring powder.
3. If food is burnt on, leave paste on overnight and wipe clean in the morning.

☐ Have your furnace cleaned and adjusted every year.

☐ Clean or replace air-conditioning filters every two months during periods of use.

☐ Research has shown that house plants help clean the indoor air. Microorganisms that live in potting soil use airborne toxins as a source of food; the plants' roots then absorb waste that the microorganisms produce. The following plants have been shown to perform this process quite efficiently when one plant is used for every 100 square feet of floor space in the home:

| | | |
|---|---|---|
| Chrysanthemum | Ivy | Philodendron |
| Dracaena | Palm | Snake plant |
| Fern | Peace lily | Spider plant |
| Gerbena daisy | | |

☐ A test kit that evaluates volatile chemical vapor contaminants (nitrogen dioxide, sulfur dioxide, trichlorethylene, perchloroethylene, toluene, chlorine, hydrogen sulfide) is available from the following company (cost is $149.95).

Nontoxic Environments
6135 Northwest Mountain View Drive
Corvallis, OR 97330
(503) 745-7838

☐ Keep children safe from potentially dangerous substances (lead, asbestos, toxic solvents) found in many art and craft supplies. Look for products bearing one of the safety seals of the Art and Craft Materials Institute. The *CP Nontoxic* seal means the product has passed safety tests. The *AP Nontoxic* seal signifies the item has passed safety, quality, and performance tests. Materials with the code *ASTM D-4236* means the product has been certified nontoxic by the Consumer Product Safety Commission.

For the definitive list of approved nontoxic art and craft supplies that are acceptable for grades K–6, send your request along with $5.00 (a well-spent investment) to:

Center for Safety in the Arts
5 Beekman Street – 10th Floor
New York, NY 10038
(212) 227-6220

☐ Air filters can be used to reduce pollutants in the home, but they will not entirely remove pollutants that continue to be released from a household source such as a wall-to-wall carpet. Removing pollutants often means removing the polluting source.

Air-filtration systems should be designed to remove both volatile chemical gasses (produced by formaldehyde, solvents, paints, pesticides, plastics, etc.) and particulates (pollen, dust, mold, dander, etc.) from the air in your home. Air filters and air-purification systems are available from:

The Allergy Store
PO Box 2555
Sebastopol, CA 95473
(800) 824-7163
(707) 823-6202
*Car air-filtration system also available.*

Berner Air Products, Inc.
PO Box 5410
New Castle, PA 16105
(800) 825-5015

EcoSource Products
PO Box 1656
Sebastopol, CA 95473
(800) 274-7040

E.L. Foust Company
PO Box 105
Elmhurst, IL 60126
(800) 225-9549
(708) 834-4952
*Car air-filtration system also available.*

Great American Filters
2107 Lawn Avenue
Cincinnati, OH 45212
(513) 731-9991
(800) 743-9991

Molly Industries
916 Briarwood Court
Mason, OH 45040
(800) 828-1945
(513) 398-8869

NEEDS
Suite 12A
527 Charles Avenue
Syracuse, NY 13209
(800) 634-1380
(315) 488-6300
*Car air-filtration system also available.*

Nontoxic Environments
6135 NW Mountain View Dr.
Corvallis, OR 97330
(503) 745-7838
*Car air-filtration system also available.*

☐ The following books are excellent sources of information on ways to combat indoor air pollution:

*Healthful Houses: How to Design and Build Your Own* by Clint Good and Debra Lynn Dadd. Bethesda, MD: Guaranty Press, 1988.

*The Healthy Home: How to Buy One, How to Build One, How to Cure a Sick One* by John Bower. Secaucus, NJ: Lyle Stuart, 1989.

*Nontoxic, Natural and Earthwise* by Debra Lynn Dadd. Los Angeles: Jeremy P. Tarcher, Inc., 1990.

*Your Home, Your Health and Well-Being* by David Rousseau , W. J. Rea, and Jean Enright. Berkeley, CA: Ten Speed Press, 1988.

## HOW TO GET MORE INVOLVED

Once you are aware of the dangers of indoor pollution and you have lessened the risks in your own home, there are other ways you can help on a broader scale.

☐ Support the following non-profit organizations that work to protect the public from hazardous household problems. (Additional information on the organizations is found beginning on page 269.)

Household Hazardous
  Waste Program
PO Box 108
Springfield, MO 65804
(417) 836-5777

National Center for
  Environmental Health
  Strategies
1100 Rural Avenue
Voorhees, NJ 08043
(609) 429-5358

The National Toxics
  Campaign
1168 Commonwealth Avenue
Boston, MA 02134
(617) 232-0327

# Chapter 17

# LEAD

The United States Department of Housing and Urban Development (HUD) estimates that 74 percent of all private housing built before 1980 contains some lead paint. According to the Centers for Disease Control (CDC), 3 million tons of old lead paint line the walls and fixtures of 57 million American homes. And the United States Public Health Service reports that one in nine children under age six have toxic lead levels in their blood.

Most homes built before 1950 contain lead paint but so do some newer homes. Most of this lead paint is found on exterior walls and trim, indoor stair trim, and radiators. Frequently, lead paint is found on indoor window and door trims, and occasionally on interior walls.

In addition to lead paint and lead-paint dust, there are other sources of lead exposure. These sources include food (airborne lead falls on agricultural areas); industrial emissions, particularly from iron and steel production and uranium mining (radon gas decays into lead); water pipes; lead-lined or soldered cans that are used for food and beverage storage; and lead-glazed ceramic and earthenware containers.

Ingested lead enters the bloodstream and moves to bones and organs. This lead can settle in body tissue for decades, and it is continuously released back into the bloodstream, causing significant cellular damage.

The Centers for Disease Control (CDC) considers 24 micrograms per deciliter of blood (mcg/dl) to be the maximum safe lead level, but a 1979 study at Harvard Medical School by Herbert Needleman, M.D., found that children with substantially lower lead levels—10–15 mcg/dl—were four times more likely to have IQ scores below 80 and seven times more likely to have learning disabilities than unexposed children. In 1991, Dr. Needleman's eleven-year follow-up report revealed that many young adults who were exposed to lead as children had behavioral problems, reading disabilities, low vocabulary test scores, poor hand-eye coordination, and a high dropout rate from school.

Lead and/or cadmium, which can cause cancer, are found in some of the glazes that are used to decorate clay and ceramics, and in some of the paint used to decorate glassware. Glazes are thin, glossy coatings; the lead in the glaze produces a shiny, smooth look, while cadmium enhances the vividness of colors. If glazes are not properly formulated, or are not fired at high enough temperatures for long enough periods, various foods, especially acidic foods, can leach toxic amounts of lead and cadmium into the food itself. When glassware is decorated with paint that contains lead, acidic beverages can leach some of the lead, which is then ingested.

Exposure to cadmium increases the risk of many forms of cancer, especially lung and prostate cancer. Exposure to lead is linked to cancer of the lung, stomach, large intestine, and kidney; it has also been known to cause birth defects.

In 1987, a widely reported case told of the near-death from lead poisoning of Seattle couple Donald and Frances Wallace. This occured over a three-year period as the result of drinking eight to ten cups of coffee daily from lead-laden mugs. The mugs, which had been purchased in Italy during a 1977 vacation, released 400 times more lead than the federal Food and Drug Administration (FDA) permitted.

The Wallace's symptoms ranged from insomnia, anemia, and dehydration, to severe abdominal cramps, sudden attacks of total body pain, weight loss, personality change, nervous-system dysfunction, and flu-like characteristics. Mr. Wallace experienced sharp pains in his wrists, which were mistakenly diagnosed as carpal tunnel syndrome. This misdiagnosis resulted in two unnecessary operations. Mrs. Wallace, after many months, was diagnosed with acute hepatic porphyria, a rare and incurable metabolic disorder.

The Wallaces discovered that most lead-poisoning victims are anemic, and that symptoms of lead poisoning, porphyria, and Alzheimer's disease are remarkably similar. Ultimately, through careful detective work, their correct self-diagnosis of acute, chronic lead poisoning (plumbism) was confirmed by doctors. While treatment cured them before the final and terminal stage of the disease, only time can measure the long-term effects.

After his experience with plumbism, Mr. Wallace founded a company (Frandon Enterprises) that markets home-use test kits to check for lead in pottery. He warns that many bright green glazes contain copper, which hastens lead release. Old bright orange glazes may contain uranium as well. In particular, orange-glazed pottery made between 1930 and 1970—some of which is prized by collectors (Fiestaware, Caliente, Early California, Harlequin, Poppytrail, Franciscanware, Jadestone, and Stonecraft Sahara)—may leach dangerous amounts of lead if the glaze is scratched.

## WHAT YOU CAN DO ON A PERSONAL LEVEL

There are many ways you can protect yourself and your family against harmful exposure to lead.

☐ The Centers for Disease Control recommends testing children for lead poisoning at age twelve months and again at twenty-four months. Make sure your doctor uses the blood-lead test, not the Free Erythrocyte Protoporphyrin (FEP) test, which is less accurate. If the level is 10–15 mcg/dl, remove all sources of lead from the child's environment and retest in three months. If it is higher than 15 mcg/dl, consult your doctor concerning treatment to remove lead from the child's body.

☐ Test your paint. If you discover that lead paint was used in your home, watch for peeling and for lead dust on windowsills, door frames, and wherever else friction may cause paint to powder. Damp mop lead dust with a high phosphate detergent or a trisodium wash. Your local health department should be able to advise you where to rent a HEPAvac (High Efficiency Particulate Air Filtered Vacuum). Do not use an ordinary vacuum because lead-dust particles pass right through its filter.

☐ It is impossible to tell by looking at glazes if they contain lead. Lead has been found in both expensive and inexpensive items. To test for lead in paint, ceramic and other glazed dishes, painted glassware, pipe solder, toys, and furniture, obtain a lead test kit (cost is approximately $25.00) from any of the following companies:

Frandon Enterprises
511 North 48th Street
Seattle, WA 98103
(800) 359-9000
(416) 293-4955

Seventh Generation
49 Hercules Drive
Colchester, VT 05446
(800) 456-1177

Hybrivet Systems
PO Box 1210
Framingham, MA 01701
(800) 262-LEAD
(508) 651-7881

☐ To remove lead paint, hire an experienced abatement contractor recommended by your health department or regional HUD office. Special equipment and protective clothing are required. Consider having doors and moldings taken out of the house for off-site paint removal. Leave your house during abatement treatment. Consider covering lead-based paint with wallpaper or other building material. If you are buying a house, have it tested for lead paint, and if there is a problem, solve it before you move in.

☐ Keep children away from areas where lead-based paint may chip, peel, or powder. A child can become lead poisoned by eating 1 milligram—equivalent to 1 gram of sugar—each day.

☐ Test your household water for lead (see Chapter 25, *Water*). A free pamphlet entitled *Lead in Your Drinking Water* is available from:

EPA Public Information Center
401 M Street, SW
Washington, DC 20460
(202) 260-2080

☐ Buy products in cans that are seamless or welded, and that have flat, black-striped seams. Some lead-soldered cans have crimped seams, and the joint line is silver-gray and irregular. Feel along the seam through the label. If the seam feels bumpy, leave the can on the shelf. Welded seams feel smooth and even, and the metal around the seams is shiny. (You can see the seam between the label and top or bottom rim of the can.)

☐ Some foods and beverages come in cans that are labeled "lead-free." Look for these products in natural foods stores.

☐ If you drink wine from a bottle with a lead-foil cap, wipe the cork and the rim of the bottle with a cloth that has been moistened with water, lemon juice, or vinegar before pouring the wine. Otherwise, you may ingest dangerous levels of lead salts that may be stuck to the rim of the bottle (see Chapter 3, *Alcohol*).

☐ Do not eat animal fats. Lead ingested by animals accumulates in their fat. When you eat animal fat, you ingest any lead that it contains.

☐ If you discover lead in your home water supply and decide to install a water filter, be sure to buy a filter that specifically removes lead. Always use cold tap water for drinking and cooking, since hot water is more likely to leach lead from pipes. Grains and vegetables cooked in lead-contaminated water can absorb as much as 80 percent of the water's lead. (Additional information on home water-filter systems is found in Chapter 25, *Water*.)

☐ Use glass (not ceramic) containers to store acidic foods (fruit, tomatoes, tomato sauces, juices).

☐ Protect children from lead (and other potentially hazardous substances) found in many art and craft supplies. Lead is a common ingredient in some oil-based paints. Choose products bearing one of the safety seals of the Art and Craft Materials Institute. The *CP Nontoxic* seal means the product has passed safety tests. The *AP Nontoxic* seal signifies the item has passed safety, quality, and performance tests. Materials with the code *ASTM D-4236* means the product has been certified nontoxic by the Consumer Product Safety Commission.

For the definitive list of approved nontoxic art and craft supplies that are acceptable for grades K–6, send your request along with $5.00 (a well-spent investment) to:

Center for Safety in the Arts
5 Beekman Street – 10th Floor
New York, NY 10038
(212) 227-6220

☐ Do not use vividly colored potteryware unless it has been tested for lead.

☐ Do not store food or beverages in antiques or collectibles.

☐ Do not use ceramic dishes made by amateurs or hobbyists.

☐ Never put earthenware in the dishwasher unless it is marked "dishwasher safe." Do not remove food stains from earthenware products with wire brushes or steel pads; this can disturb the glaze, releasing lead.

☐ If the inside of a ceramic container starts to pit or deteriorate, stop using it.

☐ If you re-use plastic bags that are painted with a store's or a manufacturer's name or logo, do not turn the bags inside out to store food in them. The paint used on the bag's label usually contains lead that can leach into the food. In testing at the University of Medicine and Dentistry of New Jersey, seventeen out of eighteen plastic bread bags were found to contain lead in the label's paint.

☐ Legumes, beans, sea vegetables (arame, nori, hijiki, kombu), vitamin C, and pectin can help protect against lead toxicity by protecting muscle tissue from lead damage, and by helping eliminate lead from the body.

## HOW TO GET MORE INVOLVED

If you are concerned about the health hazards resulting from lead and would like to become more involved, read the following suggestions.

☐ Write to companies who sell edible products in lead-soldered cans. Ask them to coat their cans with enamel. Enamel seals the can and helps protect its contents from lead.

☐ Contact the following organization, which keeps the public informed on issues concerning lead.

Physicians for Social Responsibility
1000 16th Street, NW
Washington, DC 20036
(202) 785-3771

# Chapter 18

# NUCLEAR WASTE

Nuclear waste is the nation's radioactive garbage. It is produced at hundreds of facilities across the country: nuclear power plants, nuclear weapons plants, uranium mills, factories, medical-research institutions, pharmaceutical companies, hospitals, and food and medical equipment irradiation plants.

The Department of Energy (DOE), formerly the Atomic Energy Commission, defines various radioactive waste levels. High-level waste, some of which remains radioactive for millions of years, primarily comes from spent nuclear fuel. Reprocessing wastes and mill tailings from uranium mining are also considered high-level radioactive materials. These materials are laden with strontium-90, cesium-137, and plutonium-239. Transuranic waste, which is produced by nuclear weapons plants and nuclear reactors, is radioactive material that is heavier than uranium, and includes plutonium, curium, americum, and neptunium.

Low-level waste, which is less radioactive and which was dumped at sea until the 1960s, is also produced largely by nuclear power plants. Low-level waste includes laboratory animal carcasses, irradiated reactor components, residues from the manufacturing of luminous watches, contaminated trucks and other equipment, contaminated filters from reactor cooling systems, laboratory coats and other clothing, contaminated paper products, and liquid waste that has been solidified in concrete.

The last category of nuclear waste is known as BRC, below regulatory concern. The DOE does not consider BRC waste to be hazardous enough to warrant alarm.

Radiation exposure has been linked to birth defects, genetic mutations, and virtually all types of cancer, especially leukemia and cancers of the bone, lung, and thyroid. According to John Gofman, M.D., discoverer of uranium-233 and a member of the Committee for Nuclear Responsibility in San Francisco, when cells in the body are exposed to high-level radiation, many cells in their entirety are killed before they are able to replicate themselves. Low-level radiation exposure actually induces more cancer per unit of dose. Cells that are exposed to low-level radiation undergo chromosome damage and are altered, but they are still able to reproduce, initiating the cancer process.

There are three major types of radiation emissions responsible for health problems: alpha particles, beta particles, and gamma rays. Alpha and beta particles cannot pass through the body's outer layer of dead skin; they have to be inhaled, ingested, or taken into the body through an open wound in order to cause cellular damage. Gamma rays, however, are extremely penetrating, and can easily pass through lead, concrete, and the human body.

When alpha and beta particles are taken into the body (through air, water, food, or an open wound), they may remain in the body for minutes or for a lifetime, depending on the specific radionuclide (radioactive species of an atom) present, and its chemical form. Inside the body, radionuclides may travel to bone, muscle tissue, or any specific organ. Where long-lasting radionuclides lodge is where health effects will appear.

Among nuclear waste-producing facilities are one nuclear test site and sixteen weapons sites that deal with radioactive materials. They are:

Bendix Plant, Kansas City, MO
Feed Materials Production Center, Fernald, OH
Hanford Reservation, Richland, WA
Idaho National Engineering Lab, Arco, ID
Lawrence Livermore National Laboratory, Livermore, CA

Los Alamos National Laboratory, Los Alamos, NM
Mound Laboratories, Miamisburg, OH
Nevada Test Site, Mercury, NV
Oak Ridge Reservation National Laboratory and Y-12
  Plant, Oak Ridge, TN
Paducah Gaseous Diffusion Plant, Paducah, KY
Pantex Plant, Amarillo, TX
Pinellas Plant, Largo, FL
Portsmouth Uranium Enrichment Complex, Piketon, OH
Reactive Metals, Inc., Ashtabula, OH
Rocky Flats Plant, Golden, CO
Sandia National Laboratories, Albuquerque, NM and
  Livermore, CA
Savannah River Plant, Aiken, SC

The Radioactive Waste Campaign's 1988 report entitled *Deadly Defense: Military Radioactive Landfills* revealed that at many of these nuclear waste producing locations, large quantities of tritium, uranium, plutonium, and other radioactive gases are routinely vented into the atmosphere. Liquid radioactive wastes are dumped into unlined trenches and settling ponds that sometimes overflow. When heavy rainfall increases surface runoff, the radioactive waste flows into surface waters, underground streams, and underground waterbearing rock formations known as *aquifers.*

While pollution controls may be able to control radioactive air pollution, contamination that leaks into the earth is extraordinarily difficult to stop. Once this radioactive waste contaminates water, the water cannot be made pure again.

At the Savannah River Plant, 30 million gallons of radioactive liquids are discharged into the ground each year. Near the Hanford Reservation, the Columbia River shows increasing levels of radioactivity. The Nevada Test Site has polluted the groundwater near Death Valley National Park. Water supplies of some entire cities are at risk. The Great Miami Aquifer has endangered the water supply of Cincinnati, Ohio, while the Tuscaloosa Aquifer has polluted the Atlanta, Georgia water supply.

Allegedly for national security reasons, the DOE facilities operated in virtual secrecy until the late 1980s. They were not subject to the same licensing or environmental protection regulations as commercial power reactors.

Figure 18.1 shows the locations of commercial and military nuclear facilities in the United States. Many people who live close to weapons plants and commercial reactors are deeply concerned about radioactive contamination, and with good reason. Following a fire at the Rocky Flats Plant in Golden, Colorado, plutonium levels were 400 to 1,500 times higher than their normal levels—higher than the plutonium level at Nagasaki after the bomb was dropped on Japan.

In a series of more than 100 articles in the *New York Times* begun in 1987, Keith Schneider revealed a shocking situation in the nation's nuclear-weapons plants: gross mismanagement and dangerous practices that endangered plant workers' lives and threatened entire communities. An ensuing congressional investigation confirmed that over many years, DOE had covered up countless nuclear accidents and breaches of safety regulations. As the scope of the cover-up was revealed, Senator John Glenn remarked, "We are poisoning our people in the name of national security."

In 1991, the *British Medical Journal* reported results of a study conducted on family members of workers in the Sellafield, England nuclear power plant. The Sellafield study concluded that children who were conceived after their fathers had been exposed to a total radiation dose of 10 rems over six to seven years, or one rem in the six-month period immediately prior to conception, had a six to eight times increased risk of developing leukemia. A 1987 report by the Regional Cancer Registry at Queen Elizabeth Medical Centre in Birmingham, England, found that "the proportion of early cancer deaths caused by fetal exposures to [background] gamma-radiation could lie between 66 and 96 percent."

In the United States, a study by the Columbia School of Public Health, published in 1990 in the *International Journal of Epidemiology,* found a significant association between background radiation and childhood cancers within ten miles of the

Three Mile Island nuclear facility. In 1991, the Childhood Cancer Research Institute reported a more than two times greater risk of leukemia in children living within ten miles of the Pilgrim Nuclear Power Station, and a 50 percent risk to those children who lived between ten and twenty miles from the plant.

Studies on nuclear-plant workers were conducted by the Childhood Cancer Research Institute from 1976 to 1991. Workers at the Oak Ridge Reservation National Laboratory in Oak Ridge, Tennessee, were found to have a significantly high incidence of leukemia; prostate, pancreatic, and brain cancers; lymphoma; and Hodgkin's disease. Workers at the Hanford Reservation in Richland, Washington, were observed to have a statistical significance of myeloma, lung cancer, and all female cancers. At the Savannah River Plant in Aiken, South Carolina, high rates of pancreatic cancer, leukemia, aleukemia, and other lymphatic cancers were observed among workers. At the Rocky Flats Plant in Golden, Colorado, significant findings included cases of brain tumors, liver cancer, lymphosarcoma, reticulosarcoma, myeloid leukemia, and multiple myelomas.

Cancer risks among workers at nuclear plants are elevated not only in cases where exposure doses are high, but also among workers exposed over time to very low levels of external radiation. In the vicinity of these plants, the general population may also be at comparable risk from long-term, low-level exposure.

Communities across the United States are also concerned about the transportation of nuclear materials. Radioactive materials are shipped by rail and highways to laboratories, medical facilities, military bases, and nuclear power plants. Nuclear waste is transported to disposal sites. Many communities have banned nuclear transport within their boundaries. Citizen Action reported that the number of spills from rail cars increased 46 percent between 1985 and 1991. In 1990 alone, 1,228 rail and 7,214 highway incidents resulted in the accidental release of hazardous materials and over $33 million in damages. Most road accidents occured due to the same causes that produce non-nuclear accidents: careless driving, driver fatigue, poor road conditions, excessive speed, and deer or elk on the highway at night.

**Figure 18.1**  Commercial and Military Nuclear Facilities in the
United States

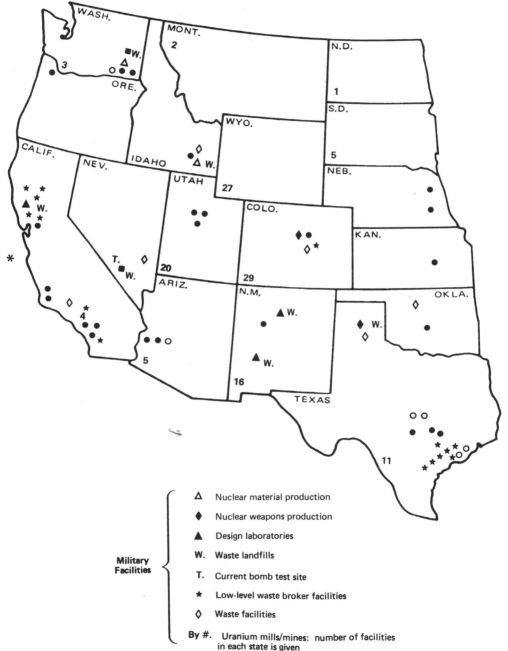

Military
Facilities

△    Nuclear material production

◆    Nuclear weapons production

▲    Design laboratories

W.   Waste landfills

T.   Current bomb test site

★    Low-level waste broker facilities

◊    Waste facilities

By #.  Uranium mills/mines:  number of facilities
       in each state is given

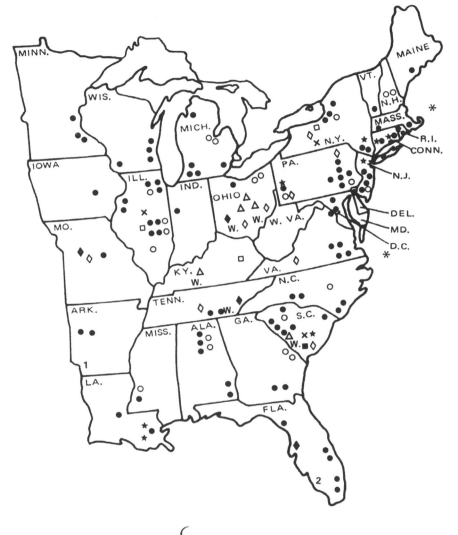

**Nuclear Power Plants, Storage and Waste Sites**

●   Operating reactors (including operating high-level waste sites)

○   Reactors under construction

■   Operating low-level waste sites

□   Closed low-level waste sites

✕   Away-from-reactor spent fuel storage sites

✳   Sea disposal sites (pre-1970)

## WHAT YOU CAN DO ON A PERSONAL LEVEL

If you live near a nuclear facility, or if you discover that nuclear waste is being transported through your community, make sure to do the following.

☐ Join a local environmental group to keep informed of what problems exist at the nuclear site, and learn how you can help avert future problems.

☐ Organize a grass-roots effort to ban the transporting of hazardous waste in your community.

## HOW TO GET MORE INVOLVED

Whether you live near a nuclear facility or not, there are ways you can effectively show your concern regarding their dangers.

☐ Write to your legislators and demand proper regulation and monitoring of all nuclear sites. Urge that epidemiological studies be performed on site workers as well as on people in surrounding communities.

☐ Support the following consumer organizations, which gather information on nuclear waste, lobby for stricter controls, and keep a watchful eye on government policies. (Additional information on the organizations is found beginning on page 269.)

Citizens Clearinghouse
  for Hazardous Waste
PO Box 6086
Falls Church, VA 22040
(703) 237-CCHW

Nuclear Free America
325 East 25th Street
Baltimore, MD 21218
(301) 235-3575

Nuclear Information and
  Resource Service
1616 P Street, NW
Washington, DC 20036
(202) 328-0002

Physicians for Social
  Responsibility
1000 16th Street, NW
Washington, DC 20036
(202) 785-3771

Radioactive Waste Campaign
7 West Street
Warwick, NY 10990
(914) 986-1115
(718) 387-8786

SANE/FREEZE
Suite 640
1819 H Street, NW
Washington, DC 20006-3603
(202) 862-9740

# Chapter 19

# OUTDOOR HAZARDS

According to the American Lung Association, 158 million people in 182 urban areas in the United States breathe air that the Environmental Protection Agency (EPA) considers unhealthy. Millions more live near, work in, or visit these metropolitan centers. Air pollution is caused by carbon monoxide and diesel particulates from motor vehicles (uncontrolled diesels can emit 30 to 100 times more particulates than gas-powered engines); oxides of sulfur and nitrogen from power plants; man-made ozone from industrial processes and mobile sources (automobiles, power boats, lawn mowers, etc.); toxic pollutants from sources as diverse as dry cleaners, auto-body paint shops, gas stations, and large industries; and weather conditions that sometimes trap pollutants close to the ground.

Each year, we breathe in millions of pounds of cancer-causing chemicals that have been released into the air, including arsenic, benzene, trichloroethylene, and vinyl chloride. Ground-level ozone, a major component of smog, is formed when pollutants combine with oxides of nitrogen in the presence of sunlight. Unfortunately, harmful ozone at ground level does not move up to replenish the deteriorating ozone layer eighteen to thirty miles above the Earth.

The upper-ozone layer is being eroded by a number of chlorine and bromine-based chemicals that are released into the atmosphere including chlorofluorocarbons (CFCs), hydrochlorofluorocarbons (HCFCs), halons (potent, ozone-depleting compounds used primarily in fire extinguishers), carbon tetrachloride, methyl chloroform (a chemical used in solvents and adhesives), and methyl bromide (an insecticide). This erosion process is accelerated by hot, sunny days, which are becoming more prevalent as trapped gases warm the Earth's atmosphere.

Over Antarctica, the ozone layer is not merely thinning, it has disappeared altogether. This phenomenon is known as the ozone hole. Because depletion of the ozone layer is not uniform, some geographical areas, such as Australia (the most populated land mass near the Antarctic ozone hole), receive a great deal more radiation than others.

In 1991, National Aeronautics and Space Administration (NASA) scientists reported that ozone depletion was no longer predominantly over the Earth's polar extremes. Densely-populated regions were being affected as well. Depletion occurs not just in winter, as had been previously believed, but in the summer as well.

In 1991, ozone depletion over the northern hemisphere was measured at more than twice the level NASA had expected a year earlier. As a result, EPA administrator William Reilly predicted that skin-cancer deaths over the next fifty years will increase to 200,000, a level 20 times greater than the 9,300 skin-cancer deaths the EPA predicted in 1988 for the same period.

The most dangerous exposure to the sun occurs during childhood years. Heavy sun exposure during childhood increases the incidence of melanoma, the most serious and potentially life-threatening skin cancer.

At a hearing in November 1991, held by Senator Al Gore, chairman of the United States Senate Commerce, Science and Transportation Committee, marine scientists revealed that because of the severe ozone depletion over Antarctica, ultraviolet radiation has deeply penetrated the ocean. This penetrating radiation has caused genetic damage in and has reduced the productivity of *phytoplankton* (single-cell organisms that form the base of the food chain). Since most of the Earth's oxygen and much of its food is supplied by the oceans, damage to marine organisms may produce effects that will ripple through all of the Earth's ecosystems.

"Non-essential" CFCs were banned in 1978 for use in spray cans but are still used in refrigerators, industrial solvents, and insulating material. The bubbles in plastic foam, leaks in defective or abandoned refrigerators, and solvents (especially those that clean computer circuits and other electronic equipment) continue to release CFCs into the atmosphere.

The landmark international agreement known as The Montreal Protocol on Substances that Deplete the Ozone Layer, drafted in 1987 and strengthened in 1990, calls for a global ban on CFCs and halons by the year 2000. Also included is a ban on the cleaning solvents carbon tetrachloride and methyl chloroform by the years 2000 and 2005, respectively. Some countries, anxious for a faster phaseout, have passed even more stringent laws. CFC production will be banned in Germany by 1995 and in Canada by 1997; Australia, Sweden, and Norway will ban halons as of 1995; and Canada will not permit the use of methyl chloroform after the year 2000.

The chemical stability of CFCs, which has made them so appealing to industry for decades, is what makes them so harmful today. Although they themselves don't break down chemically for many years, they do break down the chemistry of the upper atmosphere.

Consequently, the depleted ozone shield can no longer protect us by absorbing ultraviolet (UV) radiation. As a result, not only do thousands of cases of skin cancer appear each year, but millions of plants, trees, animals, crops, and tiny ocean organisms are damaged or killed.

It will take generations to slow down this process. Gases being released today will reach the stratosphere in seven to ten years. These gases will remain there, six to fifteen miles above the Earth's surface, for at least 100 years. Levels of ultraviolet radiation from ozone depletion will not peak until approximately 2020. If we act now to prevent further erosion of the ozone hole over Antarctica, the hole will still not be closed until—at the earliest—the year 2075.

## WHAT YOU CAN DO ON A PERSONAL LEVEL

To lower your risk against the harmful effects of outdoor pollutants and dangerous ultraviolet rays, consider the following suggestions.

□  Avoid the sun between 10 a.m. and 2 p.m.(11 a.m. and 3 p.m. daylight savings time).

□  If you are taking medication, check with your doctor to see if the medication will cause you to be extra sensitive to the sun.

□  Use a protective sunscreen with, at the very least, a 15 sunscreen protection factor (SPF). For more information on sunscreens, see the inset on page 157.

□  Studies at the University of Arizona College of Medicine and Cancer Center in Tucson indicate that di-alpha-tocopherol vitamin-E oil (but not acetate vitamin-E cream) applied to the skin protects against UV-B rays.

□  Be particularly careful in the South or Southwest, where skin-cancer rates are twice as high as in other areas of the United States.

□  Be aware that sensitivity to the sun's rays is more common for those who have fair skin that burns without tanning or that tans less than average.

□  Do not go to tanning parlors; they use UV-A light.

□  Wear sunglasses that have been coated specifically to filter UV rays.

□  Only buy new refrigerators or air conditioners that have been made with HCFC-22 (hydrochlorofluorocarbon-22) insulation, not CFC-12. HCFC-22, a transitional compound, which itself will be banned in 1994, contains only 2–10 percent of the ozone-depleting properties of CFC-12.

□  By 1995, refrigerators must be drained of coolant before being discarded. If you discard one before 1995, ask a local service shop to recycle the coolant. If you have a Whirlpool refrigerator, call (800) 253-1301 for information on coolant recycling.
 Coolant recycling will become increasingly available as manufacturers develop collection and processing programs, so check with the manufacturer of your refrigerator to learn whether they have established a coolant-recycling program.

# Know Your SPFs

*Before the 1990s, most sunscreens were formulated to block ultraviolet-B (UV-B) radiation. It is now known that ultraviolet-A (UV-A) rays also cause skin cancer. Most products with sunscreen protection factors (SPF) of 15 or more now protect against both UV-A and UV-B rays, according to Vincent A. DeLeo, M.D., director of Environmental Dermatology at New York's Columbia-Presbyterian Medical Center. Sun blocks should be used year-round, because UV-A radiation does not diminish in winter. Sunscreen should be used even on overcast days, because 80 percent of the sun's rays pass through clouds.*

*To determine how long a sunscreen will protect you, multiply the SPF by the time it usually takes you to burn. For example, if you normally burn in 20 minutes, an SPF of 15 will give you 300 minutes (or 5 hours) of protection.*

*While wearing suncreen, if you swim or perspire (e.g. during vigorous exercise), check the label to see if the sunscreen is waterproof. Reapply if necessary.*

☐ If your car air conditioner, home air conditioner, or refrigerator needs repair, look for a service center that recycles CFCs. By the end of 1992, all service centers must recycle CFCs.

☐ Do not buy halon fire extinguishers. If you have a halon extinguisher, store it until a halon reclaiming or recycling program is developed.

☐ Do not use foam building insulation, which is made with CFCs. Consider using cellulose insulation instead.

☐ Many consumer products such as insect sprays, fabric protectors, spot removers, and cleaning fluids contain methyl chloroform, also known as 1,1,1-trichloroethane. Check the labels on these products to be sure they do not contain these harmful ingredients. Look for nontoxic alternatives.

☐ Never use carbon tetrachloride or any solvents or cleaning fluids that contain this ozone-damaging chemical.

☐ For more information, read:

*Design for a Liveable Planet: How You Can Help Clean Up the Environment,* by John Naar. New York: Harper & Row, 1990.

*Our Drowning World: Population, Pollution and Future Weather,* by Anthony Milne. Garden City Park, NY: Prism Press, 1989.

**HOW TO GET MORE INVOLVED**

In addition to the suggestions presented in the previous section of this chapter, you can become more actively involved in helping protect the environment.

☐ Write letters to state and federal legislators and urge them to establish more stringent nationwide standards to reduce air pollution.

☐ Support the efforts of environmental activist groups. The following organizations are committed to helping clean up and protect our atmosphere. (Additional information on the organizations is found beginning on page 269.)

American Lung Association
1740 Broadway
New York, NY 10019
(212) 315-8700

Environmental Action
6930 Carroll Avenue
Tacoma Park, MD 20912
(301) 891-1100

Clean Water Action
Suite 300
1320 18th Street, NW
Washington, DC 20036
(202) 457-1286

Environmental Defense
 Fund
275 Park Avenue South
New York, NY 10010
(212) 505-2100

Friends of the Earth
218 D Street, SE
Washington, DC 20003
(202) 544-2600

Greenpeace International
1436 U Street, NW
Washington, DC 20009
(202) 462-1177

Natural Resources Defense
  Council
40 West 20th Street
New York, NY 10011
(212) 727-2700

Renew America
Suite 710
1400 16th Street, NW
Washington, DC 20036
(202) 232-2252

Sierra Club
730 Polk Street
San Francisco, CA 94109
(415) 923-5653

Worldwatch Institute
1776 Massachusetts Avenue
Washington, DC 20036
(202) 452-1999

# Chapter 20

# PESTICIDES IN THE HOME AND YARD

Pesticides are used in the home to control fungus, rodents, bacteria, and insects, especially termites, moths, fleas, ticks, and ants. Pesticides are used outdoors to control weeds and plant infestation. Many of these pesticides cause cancer and can be fatal if swallowed, spilled on the skin, or inhaled. Once applied, pesticides can last indoors for years; they can cause nausea, respiratory difficulties, depression, dizziness, weakness, blurred vision, tremors, and convulsions. Damage to the lungs, liver, kidneys, and heart; a suppressed immune system; sexual dysfunction; paralysis; and coma are possible results of pesticide poisoning.

Homeowners spray more pesticides on their lawns per acre than farmers do on their crops. At a 1991 Senate Environment and Public Works Subcommittee hearing, a former concert pianist and champion ice skater from River Grove, Illinois, testified to the hazardous results of pesticide use. In 1985, she was lying in her back yard when a lawn-care company sprayed her neighbor's property. The spray drifted to her yard, soaking her, her dog, and her cat. The cat died within minutes and the dog died the next day. She became ill, collapsed within minutes, and is now legally blind in one eye and permanently disabled.

Children and people on medication may be more sensitive to pesticides than other people and more susceptible to pesticide poisoning. Tom Latimer, a thirty-six-year old engineer from Dallas, Texas, testified to his near-fatal reaction to diazinon, a pesticide that had been used on his lawn. Latimer had been taking the ulcer drug Tagamet when he was exposed to diazinon as he mowed his lawn and picked up grass clippings in the spring and summer of 1985. The pesticide built up in his body and interacted with the Tagamet.

One afternoon in the late summer, as he was edging walkways and gathering grass clippings, he began to feel dizzy and nauseous. He developed a severe headache, a runny nose, and a feeling of tightness in his chest. His eyes began to jerk uncontrollably.

In November 1985, Latimer developed testicular cancer. He went through a series of tests that included liver biopsies, CAT scans, spinal-fluid taps, radioactive brain-blood flow studies, and sleep-disorder studies. Thomas Lee Kurt, a nationally recognized toxicologist, diagnosed Latimer's condition as "enhanced organophosphate (pesticide) toxicity due to Tagamet," which inhibited the metabolism of diazinon. Impaired vision, slowed speech, and a constant loss of train of thought also characterized Latimer's condition.

Heavy pesticide exposure that results in an acute toxicity syndrome such as Latimer's is not the only problem. Research shows that low-level pesticide exposure over time increases the risk of cancer, birth defects, and damage to the kidneys, liver, and nervous system.

Between 1989 and 1991, four members of the Ladies Professional Golf Association (Heather Farr, Kathy Ahern, Suzanne Jackson, and Shelley Hamlin) developed breast cancer. According to Dr. Melvin Reuber of the National Coalition Against the Misuse of Pesticides (NCAMP), 10 herbicides used on golf courses are known carcinogens. Most professional golfers have been exposed to these chemicals for decades; the problem is compounded because pesticides may interact with each other, producing exponentially higher risks to health.

The herbicide 2,4-D (also known as 2,4-D acid or 2,4-dichlorophenoxyacetic acid) was a major ingredient found in the compound Agent Orange, which was used in Vietnam. Commonly used on golf courses, lawns, and in parks, 2,4-D has caused breast cancer in animal studies on rats. In 1991, the *Journal of the National Cancer Institute* reported that dogs whose owners use 2,4-D on their lawns four or more times a year have twice as high a risk of developing lymphoma (lymphatic cancer). 2,4-D can be ingested when dogs lick their coats after walking, lying, or rolling on treated lawns, or when they eat treated grass.

## WHAT YOU CAN DO ON A PERSONAL LEVEL

The following suggestions are offered to help lower your risks against the dangerous effects of commonly used house and yard pesticides.

☐ Try every nontoxic alternative before using pesticides in your home or yard. Look for biological products such as *Bacillus thuringiensis*, which controls gypsy moths and other bugs.

☐ Make certain wooden building materials do not come into contact with the soil. This simple act will help prevent termite infestation.

☐ Store firewood away from your home to prevent termite damage. Termites have long wings, which they eventually shed, causing them to resemble ants. To avoid becoming dehydrated, some termites nest in the ground, which contains moisture, and then they tunnel to a building's foundation. In warm climates where there is constant high temperature and relative humidity, such as in southern California, Florida, and on the Gulf and southern East Coasts, termites nest in the wood itself.

☐ Exterminators commonly treat subterranean termites (the kind that live in the ground) by drilling holes around the foundation of the house and through the basement floor. Toxic chemicals are then injected into these holes. However, nontoxic alternatives are available. Dry-wood termites, woodborers, and other wood-nesting termites can be killed by heating the infested area to 140°F for ten minutes, or by using an electrical charge emitted from a device called an Electro-Gun. To locate a pest-control operator in your area who uses this chemical-free treatment, contact:

Etex, Ltd.
PO Box 33160
Las Vegas, NV 89133-3160
(800) 543-5651
(702) 382-3966

☐ Always leave the house when an exterminator is treating it with chemicals. Ventilate the house well before returning to it, and keep it ventilated for several weeks or more.

☐ Instead of using mothballs or other toxic chemicals to kill moths and their larvae, use a moth deterrent, such as cedar blocks and sachets, or store clothing in cedar chests or cedar closets. Cedar is effective because of its strong scent. Lavender or any other strong scent will also work. Cedar sachets are sold in many hardware stores and home centers; they can also be purchased from the following company:

Clear Light: The Cedar Company
PO Box 551B, State Road 165
Placitas, NM 87043
(505) 867-2381

☐ When storing woolens or any clothing that has fur or feathers, be sure they are free of grease and stains, on which moths thrive.

☐ If you find moth damage, send infested items to the dry cleaner. If damage recurs, have your house exterminated to destroy nests and kill moth larvae. Again, leave your house during extermination, and ventilate it well upon returning.

☐ Be aware that DDVP (dimethyldichlorovinylphosphate)—sold in paracrystals, paranuggets, household foggers, and sprays—and PDB (paradichlorobenzene)—sold in no-pest strips, nuggets, room air fresheners, and flea collars—kill moths but are extremely toxic. These products can cause cancer in animals, as do many ingredients in the sprays sold to kill mosquitoes, ticks, fleas, hornets, ants, and other insects.

☐ If you use toxic moth-control products, use them only in trunks or other containers that can be stored in attics or detached garages, away from living areas.

☐ Instead of using chemical products, spray ants with mint tea. Sprinkle borax or chili powder at the site where ants are coming in.

☐ Spread equal parts of borax and sugar where you see cockroaches.

☐ Use a fly swatter, or repel flies with citrus peel.

☐ If field mice nest in your house, spray strong peppermint tea along baseboards where you hear them or see their droppings.

☐ Plant mint around the foundation of your house; it is a natural insect repellent.

☐ Do not use insect repellents that contain DEET (N,N-diethyl-m-toluamide), and *never* apply them directly to skin.

☐ If you are of childbearing age, the EPA warns not to use insect repellents containing ethyl hexanediol (also known as 2-ethyl-1,3- hexanediol). Ethyl hexanediol causes birth defects in animal studies, and may cause birth defects in humans as well.

☐ The following natural insect repellents are excellent nontoxic choices.

| | |
|---|---|
| *Skin So Soft* | *Beat It!* |
| Avon Products, Inc. | Naturpath |
| 9 West 57th Street | 1410 NW 13th Street |
| New York, NY 10019 | Gainesville, FL 32601 |
| (800) 858-8000 | (800) 542-4784 |
| *Repellent for mosquitoes, fleas, other bugs.* | *Liquid insect repellent; can be used by humans and pets.* |

### Bygone Bugs

Lakon Herbals
RR1 Box 4710
Montpelier, VT 05602
(802) 223-5563

*Repellent for mosquitoes and other outdoor bugs.*

### No Common Scents

Humane Alternative Products
8 Hutchins Street
Concord, NH 03301
(603) 224-1361

*Liquid insect repellent.*

### EcoSafe Skeeter Shoo

EcoSafe Products
PO Box 1177
St. Augustine, FL 32085
(800) 274-7387
(904) 824-5884

*Repellent for mosquitoes, fleas, and flies.*

### Weeds of Work

Karen's Nontoxic Products
1839 Dr. Jack Road
Conowingo, MD 21918
(800) KARENS-4
(301) 378-4621

*Natural insect repellent.*

☐ Pyrethrin, a common ingredient in home pesticides, is the crushed, dried flowers of *chrysanthemum cinerarifolium.* Harmless to humans and pets, pyrethrin kills bugs on contact. In commercial preparations, pyrethrin is often mixed with other toxic chemicals. Use pyrethrin alone or mix it with diatomaceous earth. Sprinkled on carpets and floors, pyrethrin is effective in killing ants, fleas, and roaches. Pure pyrethrin and diatomaceous earth are available from the companies listed on page 167.

☐ If you find a bug indoors, you might want to let it go without killing it. Trap it under a glass, slip a sheet of paper under the glass to keep the bug inside, take the glass outdoors, and let the bug go.

☐ Take pesticide containers (with the original label) to hazardous-waste collection sites (see *Garbage*, Chapter 14).

☐ Do not poison your lawn (and your neighborhood) or your water supply with chemicals; buy natural lawn and garden products instead. The following companies sell chemical-free pest-control products, and other nontoxic items for the lawn and garden, such as fertilizers, pyrethrin, and diatomaceous earth. Free catalogues are available upon request.

Bricker's Organic Farms
824-K Sandbar Ferry Road
Augusta, GA 30901
(706) 722-0661
(706) 724-6901

Deer Valley Farm
RD 1 Box 173
Guilford, NY 13780
(607) 764-8556

Dirt Cheap Organics
5645 Paradise Drive
Corte Madera, CA 94925
(415) 924-0369

EcoSafe Products
PO Box 1177
St. Augustine, FL 32085
(800) 274-7387
(904) 824-5884

Garden-Ville of Austin
6266 Highway 290 West
Austin, TX 78735
(512) 892-0006
(512) 892-0002

Gardeners Supply Company
128 Intervale Road
Burlington, VT 05401
(802) 863-1700

Gardens Alive!
5100 Schenley Place
Lawrenceburg, IN 47025
(812) 537-8650

Natural Gardening Co.
217 San Anselmo Avenue
San Anselmo, CA 94960
(415) 456-5060

Natural Pest Controls
8864 Little Creek Drive
Orangevale, CA 95662
(916) 726-0855

Necessary Trading Co.
PO Box 305
New Castle, VA 24127
(703) 864-5103

Ringer Corporation
9959 Valley View Road
Eden Prairie, MN 55344
(800) 654-1047

☐ If you have questions concerning the risks or benefits of specific pesticides, call the National Pesticide Telecommunications Network 24-hour hotline at (800) 858-PEST. In addition, you can order their free publication *A Citizen's Guide to Pesticides*.

☐ For further information on pesticides and their hazards, contact:

Bio-Entegral Resource Center
PO Box 7414
Berkeley, CA 94707
(510) 524-2567

☐ See Chapter 11, *Pesticides in Food*, for more information on harmful effects of pesticides.

☐ The following books are excellent sources on nontoxic pest-control suggestions:

*Bug Busters: Poison-Free Pest Control For Your House & Garden* by Bernice Lifton. Garden City Park, NY: Avery Publishing Group, 1991.

*Pest Control You Can Live With* by Debra Graff. Sterling Heights, VA: Earth Stewardship Press, 1990.

## HOW TO GET MORE INVOLVED

If you are concerned with issues on the dangers and the misuse of pesticides in the home and yard, get actively involved.

☐ Support these public-interest groups that are concerned with pesticide misuse. (Additional information on the organizations is found beginning on page 269.)

GROW
38 Llangollen Lane
Newton Square, PA 19073
(215) 353-2838

National Coalition Against
 the Misuse of Pesticides
701 E Street, SE
Washington, DC 20003
(202) 543-5450

Natural Resources
  Defense Council
40 West 20th Street
New York, NY 10011
(212) 776-2211

Northwest Coalition for
  Alternatives to Pesticides
PO Box 1393
Eugene, OR 97440
(503) 344-5044

# Chapter 21

# PET PRODUCTS

Many pet owners believe a flea-and-tick collar is an animal's second best friend. The fact is, some of these insect collars can be dangerous to both you and your pet. In March 1988, Consumers Union urged people not to use flea-and-tick collars, no-pest strips, or insecticide sprays containing vapona or DDVP (dimethyldichlorovinylphosphate) because of cancer risks. Other toxic ingredients often found in pet collars, shampoos, or sprays are piperonyl butoxide, carbamate, carbaryl, and sevin.

Many sprays and insect collars contain solvents that cause insecticides to penetrate your pet's skin, as well as your own skin when you handle your pet. These chemicals can enter the animal's bloodstream and damage its vital organs and central nervous system. Some insecticide collars also release toxic fumes. Toxicity is much greater for pets than it is for humans because of the large dose of chemicals the animals receive per pound of body weight. Furthermore, the effectiveness of flea-and-tick collars is questionable, for the only insects repelled are those found near the collar itself, not on the rest of the animal.

Commercial pet foods can contain steroids and antibiotics (in beef and poultry), pesticides (in grains), and artificial colors and preservatives that can cause cancer. Some pet foods also contain meat and bone meal from the esophagus, diaphragms, stomachs, and blood vessels of cows, goats, pigs, and sheep; fishheads; and chicken feet, feathers, and heads. This is, literally, tough stuff to digest, so the percentage of protein listed on the label might not accurately reflect how much your animal actually absorbs. The Association of American Feed Control Officials (AAFCO) sets "adequate," not optimal, standards for commercial pet foods.

Many pets are exposed to the same passive smoke, radon, formaldehyde, electromagnetic radiation, indoor and outdoor pollution, air and water impurities, and household toxins that humans are. There is no need to subject them to a toxic or inadequate diet as well.

### WHAT YOU CAN DO ON A PERSONAL LEVEL

Help protect your pet from harmful pesticides and unhealthy food additives.

☐ Do not use pesticides or insecticides on your pet until you have tried alternatives. Many natural foods stores sell nontoxic flea-and-tick collars and other nontoxic repellents.

☐ One nontoxic measure for ridding your animal of fleas is to rub its skin and coat with a mixture of one quart of water and a teaspoon of Avon *Skin-So-Soft*, available from an Avon representative or by calling Avon at (800) 858-8000. Another nontoxic alternative for getting rid of fleas is the use of a flea comb. Be aware that a flea comb must have thirty-two teeth per inch for maximum effectiveness. The Fleamaster is an excellent flea comb and is available from:

Breeders Equipment Company
PO Box 177
Flourtown, PA 19031
(215) 233-0799

☐ If your pet spends time outdoors, do not use pesticides on your lawn. Dogs that live where lawns are treated with pesticides may have a high risk of contracting canine malignant lymphoma. (For nontoxic lawn-care alternatives, see Chapter 20, *Pesticides in the Home and Yard*.)

☐ Examine your animal daily during flea-and-tick season. If you find a tick, strike a match and blow it out. Place the still-warm match head as close as possible to the tick without touching your pet's skin. The heat will make the tick back out. When the tick's head is out, grasp it firmly with tweezers, pull it out, kill it, and dab alcohol on the animal's broken skin. You can also remove an embedded tick by covering it with vaseline; the tick will back out to avoid suffocation.

☐ For fleas, sprinkle pyrethrin around your house and on your pet's bedding. Pyrethrin is the crushed, dried flowers of *chrysanthemum cinerarifolium*. Harmless to pets and humans, pyrethrin kills bugs on contact. In commercial products, pyrethrin is often mixed with pesticides or other toxic ingredients, but it can be ordered in its pure form from the companies listed on page 167.

☐ Fleas can also be controlled by sprinkling furniture and carpets with table salt, Borax, or a mixture of pyrethrin and diatomaceous earth. (If you use Borax, keep pets away from it until you vacuum or they may ingest toxic amounts.) Diatomaceous earth is available from the companies listed on page 167.

☐ Fleas and flea larvae found in carpeting and upholstered furniture can be controlled by using sodium polyborate, a natural mineral compound marketed as Rx for Fleas Plus. To locate a registered applicator in your area, call (800) 4-NO FLEA.

☐ When dogs or cats have fleas, bathe them with mild shampoos or dishwashing liquid. Insecticide shampoos are not necessary, because fleas will drown anyway. Natural flea-and-tick-control products can be found in most natural foods stores. They can also be purchased from the following companies:

Aubrey Organics
4419 N. Manhattan Avenue
Tampa, FL 33614
(800) AUBREY-H
(813) 876-4879

Natural Pet Care
2713 East Madison Avenue
Seattle, WA 98112
(800) 962-8266
(206) 329-8565

Ringer Corporation
9959 Valley View Road
Eden Prairie, MN 55344
(800) 654-1047

Wow Bow Distributors
309 Burr Road
East Northport, NY 11731
(800) 326-0230
(516) 254-6064

☐ Look for AAFCO and Natural Resources Council statements on pet foods. They recommend that dry food with normal caloric density (3.5 to 4 kilocalories per gram) should be a *minimum* of 22 percent protein by weight, and 5 percent fat by weight. Canned food should be a *minimum* of 5.5 percent protein and 1.2 percent fat by weight.

☐ Dr. Michael Fox of the Humane Society of the United States advises pet owners to add sea vegetables (arame, wakame, nori, kombu), brewers yeast, vegetable oil, and garlic to commercial pet food to ensure optimum health.

☐ Buy name-brand pet foods, or brands that are available at natural foods stores.

☐ Do not feed vegetarian formulas to any cats or to miniature, growing, or pregnant dogs. Dogs and cats are carnivores, and they need animal protein unless a specific health condition, such as kidney disease, warrants another diet.

☐ A growing number of veterinarians are practicing holistic veterinary medicine. To locate an holistic veterinarian in your area, contact:

American Holistic Veterinary Medicine Association
2214 Old Emmorton Road
Bel Air, MD 21015
(301) 569-0795

☐ If you think your pet has been poisoned, consider calling the National Animal Poison Control Center. The Center is staffed with licensed veterinarians and veterinary toxicologists. An extensive collection of cases (over 170,000) involving pesticide, drug, plant, metal, and other poisonings in food-producing and companion animals allows the staff to make specific recommendations for your animal. There is a charge for this service. Listed below are the two payment options.

- (900) 680-0000 — $2.95 per minute
- (800) 548-2423 — $30.00 per case (credit card only)

☐ The following books are excellent sources for information on preserving the health of your pet:

> *Dr. Pitcairn's Complete Guide to Natural Health for Dogs and Cats* by Richard H. Pitcairn, V.M.D., Ph.D., and Susan Hubble Pitcairn. Emmaus, PA: Rodale Books, 1982.

> *Keep Your Pets Healthy the Natural Way* by Pat Lazarus. New Canaan, CT: Keats Publishers, 1981.

## HOW TO GET MORE INVOLVED

If you are interested in becoming more active in the protection of pets, consider the following.

☐ Support the following organizations, which are dedicated to the humane treatment of animals. (Additional information on the organizations is found beginning on page 269.)

Animal Protection Institute
PO Box 22505
Sacramento, CA 95822
(916) 731-5521

People for the Ethical
   Treatment of Animals
PO Box 42516
Washington, DC 20015-0516
(301) 770-7444

# Chapter 22

# RADIATION IN THE HOME

X-rays and gamma rays (high-frequency radiation) are known as ionizing radiation. Their penetrating rays turn atoms into charged particles called ions.

Microwaves and radio waves (low-frequency radiation) have less energy and are considered non-ionizing. However, even small doses of these waves can cause genetic damage. Many scientists and researchers believe that low-frequency radiation is cumulative, and that—as with ionizing radiation—long-term exposure increases cancer risk. The density of radio waves in our electrically and electronically engineered environment today now averages 100 to 200 times higher than the natural level of radio waves that reach us from the sun.

Researchers at the University of Washington in Seattle discovered that rats exposed to long-term, low-level microwave radiation developed malignant tumors at a rate four times higher than unexposed rats. The British medical journal *Lancet* reported in 1983 that epidemiologists observed an increased leukemia rate among people employed in electrical occupations, especially telecommunications engineers. And the New York State Department of Health reported in 1986 that prolonged exposure to low-level *electromagnetic fields* (EMFs)—fields that generate both electric and magnetic radiation—may increase cancer risks among children.

Natural fields that generate both electric and magnetic radiation surround us. These fields are generated by the planets, the sun, the moon, the Earth, and by every living thing, including our own bodies. The Earth's electromagnetic field pulses at the rate of 7.83 hertz (hz), or from maximum to minimum and back at 7.83 times a second. Our bodies, on the most basic cellular level, are regulated by and attuned to the Earth's field, and they pulse at about this same rate.

Artificial electromagnetic fields pulse at a different rate, however. Almost everything connected to an electrical circuit radiates an electromagnetic field while it operates. These artificial fields pulse at a rate of 60 hz, creating low-frequency radiation. This type of radiation is emitted by electrical transformers, video display terminals (computer monitors), telephone lines, high-tension electric wires, electrical power stations, microwave ovens, radar detectors, medical diathermy machines, citizens band radios, electric blankets, toasters, ionization-type smoke detectors, hair dryers, electric drills, electric clocks, televisions, computers, refrigerators, freezers, and dimmer and photoelectric timer switches, to name a few sources.

Both the strength of the electromagnetic field and the duration of exposure can influence health. The EPA has acknowledged, for example, that people can become ill as a result of living or working near broadcast transmitters. On the other hand, the magnetic field produced by the kind of magnet that holds memos on your refrigerator door is constant, unchanging, and non-electric; it is not considered a health risk.

In 1974, Nancy Wertheimer, Ph.D., a Boulder, Colorado epidemiologist, observed that a large number of children with leukemia lived within one or two houses of electrical transformers (the black or gray cylinders—usually about the size of a garbage can—that are mounted on power poles.) These transformers step down (reduce) high-voltage electricity to the low voltage needed to operate household appliances and electric lights.

When voltage is reduced, the strength of the electric current is increased, creating a stronger magnetic field. These invisible electromagnetic fields, which had always been considered harmless, can penetrate anything, including human bodies. Wertheimer studied the relationship of EMFs to childhood cancer for several years, and in 1979, with Edward Leeper, Ph.D., published her findings in the *American Journal of Epidemiology*. She concluded that fields created by most household appliances fall significantly with distance from the appliance, but EMFs generated by power lines remain strong for hundreds of feet.

According to a 1991 study for the Electric Power Research Institute by University of California epidemiologist John Peterson, children living near power lines have a two and a half times greater risk of developing leukemia. Similar high risks were observed in children who often used hair dryers or who watched black and white televisions, which emit higher levels of radiation than color sets.

Another Wertheimer study found that pregnant women who used electric blankets (whose magnetic fields—like those of dial-faced electric clocks—may be stronger than those generated by power lines that are associated with childhood cancer) were more likely to miscarry. Other studies have shown high miscarriage rates among pregnant women who regularly use video display terminals.

According to Paul Brodeur, author of *Currents of Death: Power Lines, Computer Terminals and the Attempt to Cover Up Their Threat to Your Health*, the electric utility companies initially tried to blame household appliances, rather than their own distribution wires, for high EMF levels. By 1986, however, investigations in the United States and abroad confirmed that exposure to low-level EMFs from power lines increased the risk of childhood leukemia.

Robert O. Becker, M.D., author of *Cross Currents: The Promise of Electromedicine, the Perils of Electropollution*, states EMFs may be linked to chronic fatigue syndrome, AIDS, autism, Fragile-X syndrome, and sudden infant death syndrome. EMFs may exacerbate pre-existing conditions such as Alzheimer's disease; Parkinson's disease; mental disorders (neuroses) such as depression, phobias, antisocial personality traits, alcoholism, drug addiction, and suicide; and malignant melanoma.

Reports have also linked EMF exposure to cancer of the breast, prostate, and brain. Pending further studies, the EPA advises "Prudent avoidance," because evidence of the danger from EMFs warrants careful additional research.

Magnetic fields are measured in gauss, a unit of magnetic force. The magnetic component of EMFs tends to be low, so they are measured in milligauss (a thousandth of a gauss). Gaussmeters are used to determine the levels of EMFs both indoors and outdoors. Although magnetic-field researchers and analysts agree that there is a relationship between adverse biological effects and exposure to EMFs, they disagree on what is considered to be a safe background level (presently, no government standards have been established). On the conservative end of the spectrum, environmental scientists agree that a background level of less than 1 mG is most desirable, and a 1.5–2 mG level is a prudent threshold for taking action. In 1982, Dr. Samuel Milham, Jr. reported in the *New England Journal of Medicine* that his studies indicated an elevated risk for all cancers among children living near power lines in homes with magnetic fields at or above 2 milligauss. (More information on gaussmeters and measuring EMFs in your home or neighborhood is found on page 184.)

Radiation is also produced in the home by tungsten-halogen bulbs and some fluorescent light bulbs. Studies conducted by the Australian National Health and Medical Research Council and the National Radiological Protection Board in Britain indicate that tungsten-halogen bulbs—though they produce more light more efficiently—emit higher amounts of ultraviolet (UV) radiation than conventional incandescent bulbs release. Desk lamps have been specifically cited as dangerous sources due to the proximity of the user to the lamp.

The glass in conventional incandescent light bulbs blocks some of the harmful UV rays; but tungsten-halogen bulbs burn at high temperatures, requiring a bulb made of fused quartz, which is an efficient conductor of UV rays. The combination of the high temperatures at which tungsten-halogen bulbs burn and the fused quartz bulbs they require produces potentially dangerous levels of UV light.

Full-spectrum light bulbs are the most desirable, as they emit 30 percent fewer UV rays than standard incandescent bulbs;

they are also glare-free. In addition, they produce a "northern sunlight" effect—the best natural light source known.

All fluorescent light bulbs contain mercury, and some compact, energy-efficient fluorescent bulbs contain radioactive material in the glow switch, also known as the glow starter or glow bottle. Fluorescent bulbs that contain radioactive material are obtusely labeled "contains CiKR-85" (curies of Krypton-85, a radioactive gas), "contains CiPM-147" (curies of Promethium-147, a radioactive metal), or "contains H-3" (a radioactive isotope also known as tritium, a radioactive gas.)

These radioactive materials are released only if the bulb is broken. However, those bulbs that are not broken during usage are virtually always broken when they are disposed of in landfills, releasing mercury and radioactive material through the landfill and eventually into the water supply.

Some symptoms of exposure to non-ionizing radiation sources are muscle pain and spasms, fatigue, sleeplessness, headaches, anxiety, moderate to severe ear pain, labored breathing, heart palpitations, and nausea.

## WHAT YOU CAN DO ON A PERSONAL LEVEL

You have the power to make a difference. The following suggestions are concrete ways to reduce the odds against exposure to harmful radioactive waves and electromagnetic fields.

☐ Install shielded wire in your home. You can reduce the magnetic field that surrounds your household wiring by approximately 80 percent if you twist the wires around each other (one twist every two to three inches).

☐ Reduce exposure to radio and microwave sources. Shield sources with metal screens or aprons, and make sure microwave oven doors close securely. The government has issued standards for radiation emissions. Most manufacturers state that their products are safe and do not emit dangerous radiation levels *if they are operating properly*. However, leaks may develop over time due to manufacturing defects, the deterioration of shielding or sealing parts, or as a result of improper maintenance.

☐ Be sure all radio-wave and microwave sources are tightly sealed; reduce the time you spend close to them. Step back at least six feet from a microwave oven while it is on. This can reduce the amount of radiation you receive by 75 percent.

☐ Keep a distance of six feet from fluorescent lights. Energy-efficient fluorescent bulbs that are long-lasting, do not contain radioactive material, and do not flicker or hum—as other fluorescent bulbs tend to do—range in price from $25.00–30.00 (depending on wattage), and can be ordered from:

EcoWorks                          Seventh Generation
2326 Pickwick Road                49 Hercules Drive
Baltimore, MD 21207               Colchester, VT 05446
(301) 448-3319                    (800) 456-1177

Real Goods
966 Mazzoni Street
Ukiah, CA 95482
(800) 762-7325

☐ Do not use tungsten-halogen desk lamps. Full-spectrum incandescent light bulbs are the most desirable; they are approximately four times longer lasting than regular incandescent bulbs. At a cost of under $10.00, full-spectrum light bulbs can be ordered from:

Advanced Lighting Technology
M. Pencar Associates
137-75 Geranium Avenue
Flushing, NY 11355
(800) 788-5781
(718) 939-7031

☐ Keep a distance of four feet or more from television sets, refrigerators, and freezers; three feet from electric heaters; and at least one foot from hair dryers. Sit two-and-a-half to three feet from the front of video display terminals, and stay four feet away from the back and sides.

☐ If you have ionization-type smoke detectors, replace them with photoelectric models.

☐ Place dial-faced electric clocks at least three feet away from your bed. Other electric clocks should be at least one foot away.

☐ Get an EMF shield for your video display terminal and television set; it can reduce the magnetic field by 85 percent. The cost of these shields ranges from $40.00–200.00. They are sold in electronics stores or can be ordered from:

Langley-St. Clair, Inc.      Safe Technologies Corp.
132 West 24th Street      33 William Street
New York, NY 10011      Needham, MA 02194
(800) 221-7070      (800) 638-9121
                     (617) 444-7778

☐ Whenever possible, use battery-operated appliances rather than electrically operated devices. Batteries produce a weaker field.

☐ Install non-electric energy sources in your home, such as solar-heat panels.

☐ Do not use remote devices such as cordless and cellular telephones, or those that are used for garage doors, televisions, VCRs, or toys. Remote devices tend to generate strong EMFs.

☐ When any electrical or electronic source is not in use, turn it off and unplug it. As long as an electrical source is plugged in, the wires are "hot," and power is flowing through them.

☐ To measure the EMFs in your home or neighborhood, contact an environmental testing service or consider purchasing a gaussmeter, an easy-to-use device that measures both indoor and outdoor EMFs. The only way to know the exact field of any specific appliance is to measure it with a gaussmeter. Consider sharing the cost of buying one with your neighbors (prices start at about $100.00). If the field is high in your home, remove the devices and appliances that register elevated readings, or keep away from them as much as possible.

Gaussmeters can be purchased from:

Environmental Testing
  & Technology
PO Box 369
Encinitas, CA 92024
(619) 436-5990

Safe Technologies Corp.
33 William Street
Needham, MA 02194
(800) 638-9121
(617) 444-7778

Real Goods
966 Mazzoni Street
Ukiah, CA 95482
(800) 762-7325

Schaefer Applied
  Technology
200 Milton Street
Dedham, MA 02026
(800) 366-5500

Safe Environments
2512 Ninth Street
Berkeley, CA 94710
(800) 356-2663
(510) 549-9693

☐ Use non-electric energy products that operate by wind, water, or solar power. A full line of alternative-energy products can be ordered from:

Real Goods
966 Mazzoni Street
Ukiah, CA 95482
(800) 762-7325

Seventh Generation
49 Hercules Drive
Colchester, VT 05446
(800) 456-1177

☐ For more information on electromagnetic fields and radioactive waves (both in and out of the home), read:

*Cross Currents: The Promise of Electromedicine, the Perils of Electropollution* by Robert O. Becker, M.D. NY: St. Martin's Press, 1990.

*Currents of Death: Power Lines, Computer Terminals, and the Attempt to Cover Up Their Threat to Your Health* by Paul Brodeur. New York: Simon and Schuster, 1990.

*Radiation and Human Health* by Dr. John W. Gofman. San Francisco: Sierra Club Books, 1981.

## HOW TO GET MORE INVOLVED

If you are concerned with in-home radiation and the dangers of electromagnetic fields, there are ways you can get involved on a broader level.

☐ Write to computer manufacturers and urge them to redesign video display terminals to reduce EMF exposure.

☐ Write to the Environmental Protection Agency and to your legislators. Urge them to research the dangers of EMFs more thoroughly.

☐ Support organizations that gather up-to-date information on in-home radiation and EMFs, including the following public-interest groups. (Additional information on the groups is available beginning on page 269.)

Public Citizen
2000 P Street, NW
Washington, DC 20036
(202) 833-3000

Union of Concerned Scientists
26 Church Street
Cambridge, MA 02236
(617) 547-5552

Physicians for
  Social Responsibility
1000 16th Street, NW
Washington, DC 20036
(202) 785-3771

U.S. Public Interest
  Research Group
215 Pennsylvania Avenue, SE
Washington, DC 20003
(202) 546-9707

# Chapter 23

# RADON

Radon is a chemically inactive, colorless radioactive gas that occurs naturally. Radon results from the natural breakdown of uranium-238 in soil or rock, especially granite, shale, and phosphate. It can pass through solid materials, including buildings and the human body.

The National Cancer Institute estimates that radon causes 20,000–30,000 deaths a year. In the United States, radon is second only to tobacco as a primary cause of lung and possibly stomach cancer. Radon acts synergistically with tobacco smoke, multiplying exponentially the cancer risk for smokers when radon is present.

Environmental Protection Agency (EPA) studies indicate that as many as 10 percent of the homes (approximately 8 million) in the United States have elevated radon levels. The percentage is higher in areas with certain soil and bedrock formations. High concentrations of radon exist along the Reading Prong—a geological rock formation extending from Reading, Pennsylvania, through New Jersey, and into New York State. Radon is prevalent across North Dakota and Minnesota; in Colorado, Indiana, Kansas, Pennsylvania, Rhode Island, Wisconsin, and Wyoming; and wherever uranium mines are operated or uranium tailings (waste) are used as landfill or in cement.

In the 1970s and early 1980s, experts debated the extent of the radon problem in the United States. The EPA was spurred to define safe exposure levels in 1984, when Stanley Watrous set off radiation monitors on his way into work at the Limerick Nuclear Power Plant near Pottstown, on the Reading Prong. Testing revealed that the plant had no leaks, but Mr. Watrous' home had the highest radon level ever recorded—2,700 pCi/L (picocuries per liter of air). This level was 650 times higher than normal, which subjected the Watrous family each day to what was the equivalent of over 100 chest x-rays.

The United States Department of Energy (DOE) has targeted some radon-prone areas across the country through geological research. However, radon is unpredictable; one home may have life-threatening levels, while another, 100 feet away, may be uncontaminated.

Radon enters buildings through basement dirt floors, cracks in concrete floors and walls, drain pipes, floor drains, sumps, joints, and tiny cracks or pores in cinder-block walls. Radon can enter wells, reservoirs, and aquifers from contaminated rocks and soil. Underground water, including well water, generally has a higher radon content than surface water. Most public water supplies are drawn from surface water, and as surface water is exposed to the air, any radon that may be present generally escapes into the air before it reaches your tap.

Outdoors, radon disperses in the atmosphere. Indoors, the normal flow of air from the basement through the floors above draws radon with it, especially in some newer buildings with energy-efficient tight doors, thick windows, and dense insulation. Radon's decay products (radon "daughters"), such as polonium, lead, and bismuth, can attach electrostatically to household surfaces, and especially to tiny, respirable particles of dust and smoke. When these particles are inhaled, they lodge in the lungs and continue to release radioactive energy.

Two tests are most commonly used in detecting radon levels. One is a short-term charcoal canister test, in which a container of activated charcoal granules traps the radon. After a specified time, usually several days, the container is returned to the lab for analysis. The second test is an alpha track detector test that remains in place for several months. Radon does not always seep into buildings at a uniform rate, and a short-term reading can overstate or understate annual exposure. In the alpha track test, as radon decays, its radioactive decay products (alpha particles) strike a sheet of polycarbonate plastic in a filtered container and mark it with microscopic radiation tracks. At the end of the test period, this container is returned to a lab for results. Continuous monitors can be programmed to activate fans, blowers, dampers, or vents when radiation levels rise.

Radon is measured in picocuries per liter of air (pCi/L). Nationwide, the outdoor radon level averages 0.2–0.7 pCi/L, and the indoor level averages 1.3 pCi/L. Table 23.1 shows the radon risks for the general population. The EPA considers a reading of 3.0 to be safe, but a 4.0 reading to require action. Dr. Vernon J. Houk, Assistant Surgeon General with the United States Public Health Service, has described daily exposure to 4 picocuries as equivalent to 200–300 chest x-rays yearly, or the same as smoking ten cigarettes each day.

## WHAT YOU CAN DO ON A PERSONAL LEVEL

If you suspect the presence of radon in your home, the following suggestions will prove helpful.

☐ Have your house and water supply tested for radon. Fortunately, radon contamination can be removed once its presence has been established. The Radon Measurement Proficiency Report, a list of qualified testers, is available from your local EPA regional office or from:

EPA Public Information Center
401 M Street, SW
Washington, DC 20460
(202) 260-2080

☐ Radon test kits, which range in price from $20.00 to $40.00, are available from:

The Allergy Store
PO Box 2555
Sebastopol, CA 95473
(800) 824-7163

NEEDS
527 Charles Avenue – Suite 12A
Syracuse, NY 13209
(800) 634-1380
(315) 488-6300

## Table 23.1   Radon Risk Evaluation Chart

| Annual Radon Level | If a community of 100 people were exposed to this level: | This risk of dying from lung cancer compares to: |
| --- | --- | --- |
| 100 pCi/L | About 35 people in the community may die from Radon. | Having 2,000 chest x-rays each year |
| 40 pCi/L | About 17 people in the community may die from Radon. | Smoking 2 packs of cigarettes each day. |
| 20 pCi/L | About 9 people in the community may die from Radon. | Smoking 1 pack of cigarettes each day. |
| 10 pCi/L | About 5 people in the community may die from Radon. | Having 500 chest x-rays each year. |
| 4 pCi/L | About 2 people in the community may die from Radon. | Smoking half a pack of cigarettes each day. |
| 2 pCi/L | About 1 person in the community may die from Radon | Having 100 chest x-rays each year |

Levels as high as 3500 pCi/L have been found in some homes. The average Radon level outdoors is around .2pCi/L or less.

The risks shown in this chart are for the general population, including men and women of all ages as well as smokers and non-smokers. Children may be at higher risk.

SOURCE: Environmental Protection Agency, Radon Division, 1992.

☐ If a charcoal canister test shows that you have a high radon level, repeat the test with an alpha track detector. If a problem is confirmed, ask your state bureau of radiological health, your state or local health department, or the state department of environmental protection to refer you to a list of approved remediation contractors.

☐ Depending on the radon level and entry points, the problem can usually be solved simply by sealing cracks in basement walls and/or floors and by opening existing windows and vents. When further treatment is required, it usually involves installing or improving ventilation systems on the basement level.

☐ For more information, contact the EPA Public Information Center (address on page 189) and request the free booklets *A Citizen's Guide to Radon: What It Is and What To Do About It,* and *Radon Reduction Methods: A Homeowner's Guide.*

## HOW TO GET MORE INVOLVED

The organizations listed below are actively involved with public-interest issues including the dangers of radon. (Additional information on the organizations is found beginning on page 269.)

National Center for
  Environmental Health
  Strategies
1100 Rural Avenue
Voorhees, NJ 08043
(609) 429-5358

Physicians for Social
  Responsibility
1000 16th Street, NW
Washington, DC 20036
(202) 785-3771

# Chapter 24

# STOVES, HEATERS, AND FIREPLACES

In the wake of the 1970s energy crisis, wood-burning stoves became the politically correct alternative for people who wanted to reduce their dependence on foreign oil. As it turns out, however, in return for lower heating bills, homes were filled with organic woodsmoke compounds that were linked to lung cancer, heart disease, and disorders of the nervous system.

According to the Environmental Protection Agency (EPA), wood-burning stoves, fireplaces, and unvented space heaters emit polycyclic aromatic hydrocarbons that can cause eye, nose, and throat irritation; respiratory infections; bronchitis; and lung cancer. Other pollutants, such as carbon monoxide, nitrogen dioxide, and benzo-a-pyrene (a potent carcinogen), can be downdrafted from the flues of fireplaces and wood-burning stoves that have no outside air-supply vent, particularly in energy-efficient, weather-tight homes. These pollutants attach themselves to small respirable particles and, when inhaled, are carried deep into the lungs.

Combustion gases and particulates, including formaldehyde, various oxides, and chemical vapors are also released directly into homes by improperly installed and maintained chimneys and flues. Other sources of these gases and particulates are cracked furnace heat exchangers, unvented gas or kerosene heaters, and central forced-air gas-heat systems.

## WHAT YOU CAN DO ON A PERSONAL LEVEL

If you use a wood-burning stove, an unvented space heater, or a fireplace, the following suggestions will help lower your risks against the pollutants they emit.

☐ Have a trained professional inspect, clean, and tune up your furnace, flues, stovepipes, and fireplaces every year. Repair any cracks and leaks.

☐ Change filters on all heating and cooling systems according to manufacturers' directions, or every two months during periods of use.

☐ Choose wood-burning stoves that meet EPA emission standards. Make sure the stove doors fit securely. Newer stoves with low-heat-input pilot lights produce fewer pollutants than older stoves.

☐ Some gaskets in old wood-burning stove doors contain asbestos. Replace them with fiberglass gaskets. Instructions on how to properly replace these gaskets can be found in the free booklet *Asbestos in Your Home*, available from:

EPA Public Information Center
401 M Street, SW
Washington, DC 20460
(202) 260-2080

☐ Vent all heat sources to the outdoors. If you use an unvented space heater, make sure the room has cross ventilation. Operate space heaters according to manufacturers' instructions. A consistent yellow-tipped flame usually means the heater needs an adjustment.

☐ Burn only aged or cured wood; it creates less smoke. Do not buy pressed wood, sawdust logs, or any wrapped logs; they are pressure-treated with chemicals.

☐ Keep your house well ventilated; it is important to have a flow of air from the outside. Do not seal your home with weatherstripping, caulking, or extra insulation so that it is air-tight. Open doors and windows when weather permits. If you need more ventilation, install a heat-recovery ventilator, also called an air-to-air heat exchanger. This two-way ventilator draws outdoor air into the house and recovers the heat from the indoor air before exhausting it to the outside. A free air-to-air heat-exchanger fact sheet is available from:

Renewable Energy Information
PO Box 8900
Silver Spring, MD 20907
(800) 523-2929

☐ For an air-to-air heat exchanger that also filters incoming air and recirculated indoor air, contact:

Berner Air Products, Inc.
PO Box 5410
New Castle, PA 16105
(800) 852-5015

## HOW TO GET MORE INVOLVED

Awareness is your best tool against the pollutants created by wood-burning stoves, unvented heaters, and fireplaces.

☐ For more information on indoor air quality, contact the following agencies:

Office on Energy and
  the Environment
U.S. Department of Housing
  and Urban Development
Washington, DC 20410
(202) 708-4532

EPA Public Information
  Center
401 M Street, SW
Washington, DC 20460
(202) 260-2080

| Unit / Average Cost | How It Works | What It Does |
|---|---|---|
| Reverse Osmosis Unit $99–600 | Strains out contaminants through semipermeable, coiled plastic membranes. As water molecules are forced through the membranes, the contaminants are left behind. In most units, only 10–25 percent of the water passes through the strainer and into a holding tank. The rest is wasted, going down the drain with the removed contaminants. | Removes dissolved solids, some VOCs, THMs, and pesticides, as well as beneficial trace minerals. Most do not remove radon. |
| Carbon Block/ Reverse Osmosis Unit $350–900 | Most systems consist of three canisters: a particulate prefilter, a reverse osmosis membrane, and an activated carbon filter. Each component needs to be replaced periodically. Prefilters usually need to be changed every few months, the membranes every two to five years, and the carbon filters every year. | Removes microorganisms, VOCs, radon, THMs, pesticides, and dissolved solids . |
| Distiller Units $150–450 | Heats water until it turns to steam; the steam rises into cooling coils, circulates, and is then condensed into water again, leaving the contaminants that do not boil or evaporate behind in the boiling tank. Distillers must be cleaned every two weeks to six months. These units use more electricity than others, but parts do not need to be replaced. Glass units are preferable to stainless steel models. | Removes microorganisms, particulates, dissolved solids, and radioactive particles that are too heavy to rise with the water vapor. High water temperatures can, however, volatize THMs and radon if they are already present. |

# Chapter 25

# WATER

Household water comes from two sources: surface water, which is drawn from lakes, rivers, and streams; and groundwater, which comes from underground *aquifers* (formations of water-containing sand, gravel, and porous rock). Some water is contaminated due to specific, identifiable sources such as industrial or municipal waste pipes, chemical leaks or spills, and household drains. Contaminated water can also be the result of diffuse, hard-to-pinpoint sources such as pesticide-carrying agricultural run-off; deposits of contaminated soil in rivers after a storm; or roadtop run-off of film, salts, and motor oils. One quart of motor oil can contaminate a million gallons of water.

Each year in the United States over 70 billion gallons of hazardous waste are generated and "dumped." Much of this waste winds up seeping through the soil into both surface and groundwater. More contaminants are added from water pipes that leach lead, vinyl chloride, asbestos, cadmium, copper, and iron in toxic amounts.

According to the Center for the Study of Responsive Law's 1988 report *Troubled Waters on Tap: Organic Chemicals in Public Drinking Water Systems and the Failure of Regulation*, since the 1974 Safe Drinking Water Act was passed, 2,110 organic and inorganic contaminants have been identified in water. A total of 97 of these contaminants are known or suspected carcinogens; 82 are known or suspected mutagens, which cause birth defects; and 23 are tumor promoters. The remaining 1,880 have not yet been tested for toxicity.

Bottled water is defined by the FDA as water that "is sealed in bottles or other containers and intended for human consumption." Water that is bottled from "natural" sources is not required to be "pure" but may, in fact, come from local springs, wells, or even taps.

Companies that sell bottled water are not required to identify the water source or state the type of purification treatment used on their labels. Most bottled water is not tested for toxic chemicals, and much of it does not meet federal water-quality standards. In some states, manufacturers are required to have bottled water tested by a certified laboratory.

Depending on where you live and where your water supply comes from, household water should be tested for the following pollutants.

- *Microorganisms*, including bacteria, viruses, algae, cysts, and protozoans.
- *Particulates*, including asbestos, arsenic, barium, lead, selenium, rust, sediment, sand, and all heavy metals.
- *Dissolved solids*, including fluoride, nitrates, sulfates, and salts.
- *Radioactive particles*, including barium and radium.
- *VOCs (volatile organic compounds)*, including chlorine, pesticides, benzene, chlorinated hydrocarbons, PCBs (polychlorinated biphenyls), and THMs (trihalomethanes).

THMs, suspected of causing cancer and birth defects, are formed when organic matter in water reacts to chlorine. In some climates they are more prevalent in the fall, when decayed vegetation abounds. High temperatures vaporize THMs, turning them to gases. Exposure to THMs through skin contact in showers and through the air near operating dishwashers and washing machines can be 100 times greater than from drinking water. The higher the water temperature, the more THMs are produced.

Water testing can be expensive. Some local and state health departments test water for bacteriological contaminants, pesticide residues, and 129 EPA "priority pollutants" without charge, especially if a contaminated well has been cited in the neighborhood or there are other specific causes for concern.

Point-of-source filter systems are attached to a single water source, such as the kitchen tap to purify cooking and drinking water, or to an individual shower head to prevent the formation of THMs if the water is chlorinated. Point-of-source filter systems can also be attached to the main pump through which all household water flows. These filter systems meet most household water purification needs adequately, and they are generally less expensive than systems that are designed to purify entire household water supplies. Table 25.1 describes the different water systems available.

### Table 25.1   Water Filter Units

| Unit / Average Cost | How It Works | What It Does |
|---|---|---|
| Carbon Block Unit $99–375 | Traps contaminants in activated carbon filters. Filters need to be changed every few months to prevent trapped pollutants from being released into the water. The most efficient units have two separate canisters, one that prefilters sediment and one that filters through carbon. (Sediment filters are inexpensive, and changing them can prolong the life of the more expensive carbon filters.) | Filters microorganisms, VOCs, radon, and pesticides without removing beneficial trace elements. |

| Unit / Average Cost | How It Works | What It Does |
|---|---|---|
| Reverse Osmosis Unit $99–600 | Strains out contaminants through semipermeable, coiled plastic membranes. As water molecules are forced through the membranes, the contaminants are left behind. In most units, only 10–25 percent of the water passes through the strainer and into a holding tank. The rest is wasted, going down the drain with the removed contaminants. | Removes dissolved solids, some VOCs, THMs, and pesticides, as well as beneficial trace minerals. Most do not remove radon. |
| Carbon Block/ Reverse Osmosis Unit $350–900 | Most systems consist of three canisters: a particulate prefilter, a reverse osmosis membrane, and an activated carbon filter. Each component needs to be replaced periodically. Prefilters usually need to be changed every few months, the membranes every two to five years, and the carbon filters every year. | Removes microorganisms, VOCs, radon, THMs, pesticides, and dissolved solids . |
| Distiller Units $150–450 | Heats water until it turns to steam; the steam rises into cooling coils, circulates, and is then condensed into water again, leaving the contaminants that do not boil or evaporate behind in the boiling tank. Distillers must be cleaned every two weeks to six months. These units use more electricity than others, but parts do not need to be replaced. Glass units are preferable to stainless steel models. | Removes microorganisms, particulates, dissolved solids, and radioactive particles that are too heavy to rise with the water vapor. High water temperatures can, however, volatize THMs and radon if they are already present. |

| Unit / Average Cost | How It Works | What It Does |
|---|---|---|
| Ion-Exchange Unit (Water Softener) $750–1,200 | Filters hard water through synthetic resin beads to which sodium ions are loosely attached. As salt water from a brine tank flows through the resin, the resin gives up its hard mineral ions in exchange for soft sodium ions, and the softened water then flows to the faucets. These units are appropriate when the mineral content in household water is very high and/or when minerals are staining bath and kitchen fixtures or building up scaly deposits on water pipes and water heaters. | Eliminates hardness ions (mostly calcium and magnesium). Removes all beneficial trace minerals. |

## WHAT YOU CAN DO ON A PERSONAL LEVEL

If you are concerned with the water quality in your home, there are steps you can take to improve it.

☐ If you are served by a public water supply, ask your water utility to provide you with the results of any chemical tests they have performed. If you live near a Superfund site (see Chapter 15, *Hazardous-Waste Sites*) petition the EPA to conduct comprehensive tests in your home.

☐ If your local government health agencies do not perform water tests, order a test kit (prices begin under $100.00) from a certified independent laboratory. Test kits provide special containers along with instructions for obtaining water samples. The samples are then returned to the laboratory for analysis. It is prudent to have tests analyzed by a company that does not sell water-filter systems. The following companies provide water test kits and will help you decide what to test for, depending on where you live and where your water supply comes from. Depending on test results, the companies will advise you on possible plans of action.

National Testing Labs
6151 Wilson Mills Road
Cleveland, OH 44143
(800) 458-3330

WaterTest Corp.
PO Box 186
New London, NH 03257
(800) 426-8378

Suburban Water
  Testing Labs
4600 Kutztown Road
Temple, PA 19560
(800) 433-6595

☐ If your water is contaminated, notify your water company and your state and local health departments.

☐ Water-filter systems are available from the following companies:

Coast Filtration
142 Viking Avenue
Brea, CA 92621
(714) 990-4602

EcoSource Products
PO Box 1656
Sebastopol, CA 95473
(800) 274-7040

Culligan Company
1 Culligan Parkway
Northbrook, IL 60062
(800) 792-0092

NEEDS
527 Charles Avenue – Suite 12A
Syracuse, NY 13209
(800) 634-1380
(315)488-6300

The Ecology Box
2260 South Main Street
Ann Arbor, MI 48103
(800) 735-1371
(313) 662-9131

Nontoxic Environments
6135 NW Mountain View Dr.
Corvallis, OR 97330
(503) 745-7838

Pure Water, Inc.
PO Box 83226
Lincoln, NE 68501
(800) 842-5805

Real Goods
966 Mazzoni Street
Ukiah, CA 95482
(800) 762-7325

The Pure Water Place
PO Box 6715
Longmont, CO 80501
(303) 776-0056

Shaklee
444 Market Street
San Francisco, CA 94111
(800) SHAKLEE

☐ The following company offers a portable water-filter system. The unit weighs only 12 ounces and is perfect for travelers.

Recovery Engineering
2229 Edgewood Avenue South
Minneapolis, MN 55426
(800) 845-7873

☐ If you drink bottled water, write to the bottler and ask for test results of bacteria, chemical contaminants, chlorination by-products, heavy metals, radiological contaminants, and sodium content of their product. Ideally, drinking water should be free of chemicals and radiation, disinfected by ozone instead of by chlorine, and low in sodium content.

☐ Store and dispose of hazardous chemicals (and their containers) properly. The Clean Water Action Project—the organization responsible for drafting both the Clean Water Act and the Safe Drinking Water Act—urges that we help reduce water contamination through proper storage and disposal of all hazardous chemicals and their containers. Waste oils, batteries, acids, corrosives, pesticides, household cleaners, flammables, outdated medicines, paints, paint removers, and wood preservatives should be brought to a hazardous-waste site. If improperly disposed of (thrown into the trash or poured down the drain) these products can contaminate both ground and surface water. In addition, these chemicals can cause pipes to corrode and toxic fumes to back up into the house. (See Chapter

14, *Garbage*, for further information on proper hazardous-waste disposal.)

## HOW TO GET MORE INVOLVED

Your voice is a powerful tool in the fight for clean water. Show your concern by speaking out.

☐ If there is no hazardous-waste collection in your community, contact the following groups for help in getting a program started.

EPA Hazardous Waste
  Hotline
(800) 424-9346

League of Women Voters
(202) 429-1965

☐ If you have a question concerning the safety of your drinking water, contact:

EPA Safe Drinking Water Hotline
(800) 426-4791
(202) 382-5533

☐ Demand action from elected officials to encourage programs that protect our lakes, rivers, and oceans from industrial pollution and other forms of waste dumping.

☐ For information on how to have an impact on clean-water issues, contact the following environmental organizations. (Additional information on the organizations is found beginning on page 269.)

American Ocean
  Campaign
2219 Main Street – Suite 2B
Santa Monica, CA 90405
(310) 576-6162

Citizens Clearinghouse for
  Hazardous Waste
PO Box 6086
Falls Church, VA 22040
(703) 237-CCHW

Clean Water Action
Suite 300
1320 18th Street, NW
Washington, DC 20036
(202) 457-1286

Earth Island Institute
300 Broadway – Suite 28
San Francisco, CA 94133
(415) 788-3666

Environmental Defense
  Fund
257 Park Avenue South
New York, NY 10010
(212) 505-2100

Greenpeace International
1436 U Street, NW
Washington, DC 20077
(202) 462-1177

Natural Resources
  Defense Council
40 West 20th Street
New York, NY 10011
(212)727-2700

U.S. Public Interest
  Research Group
215 Pennsylvania Avenue, SE
Washington, DC 20003
(202) 546-9707

# Chapter 26

# X-RAYS

X-rays, first developed in 1895, have been one of modern medicine's most significant diagnostic tools. However, x-rays produce ionizing radiation that can damage tissue. Sometimes, the body is able to repair the damage, but x-rays often cause genetic changes that can lead to cancer.

Public awareness of the effects of ionizing radiation, in which penetrating rays turn atoms into charged particles called ions, was heightened in the wake of the World War II Hiroshima and Nagasaki bombings. It was then that people realized that the survivors suffered from genetic damage and greatly increased cancer risks.

Today, the medical profession is alert to the dangers of x-rays. Dosages for diagnostic tests have been reduced to a minimum, particularly for mammograms and dental x-rays. Many physicians now advise against routine x-rays in annual checkups, and the American Dental Association advises patients not to have full-mouth x-rays. The United States Department of Health and Human Services recommends that people not ask for x-rays unless a doctor or dentist recommends it. When x-rays are taken, a shield should always be used to protect the other parts of the body.

Be aware of the newer diagnostic procedures that are often currently used instead of or in conjunction with x-rays:

- *Bone Scans* are used to check the skeleton for tumors, infections, injuries, or unexplained pain. The patient is given radioisotopes (radionuclides), which are radioactive compounds used diagnostically in tracer studies. Next, the patient is placed under a gamma camera. The image produced points out areas of increased activity, which can indicate abnormalities weeks or months before they are revealed by standard x-rays. Radiation dose is less than 1 rad.

- *V-P Scanning (Ventilation-Perfusion Scintigraphy)* is used to examine the lungs, especially for embolisms. As in a bone scan, radioisotopes and a gamma camera are used for measurement. Radiation dose is approximately .5 rad.

- *CAT or CT Scans (Computerized Axial Tomography)* are used to identify tumors and to measure their size and volume. CAT scans are also used to examine internal injuries. A computer converts digital-form findings to a three-dimensional image in approximately forty seconds. Radiation dose is less than 1 rad.

- *Doppler Flow Imaging* is used to evaluate blood flow throughout the body, even in very deep vessels. An ultrasound beam produces a tracing of peaks and valleys, and can pinpoint areas of blockage in individual vessels or in all vessels simultaneously. No radiation dose is delivered.

- *DSA (Digital Subtraction Angiography)* is used to diagnose blocked arteries. A contrast dye is injected through a catheter into the blood vessel that is to be examined. An image is then produced that provides a clear outline of veins and arteries, including any trouble spots. Radiation dose is approximately 1 rad.

- *Mammography* (which produces mammograms) is used to detect breast tumors. An image is created on x-ray film. Radiation dose is approximately 2 rads for two views of both breasts.

- *PET (Positron Emission Tomography)* is used to look at metabolic activity inside organs, especially the brain and the heart. Radioactive tracer substances can study epilepsy, Parkinson's disease, Alzheimer's disease, schizophrenia, and a host of other disorders. Radiation dose is approximately .5 rad.

- *RIA (Radioimmunoassay)* is used to determine the level of various hormones, nutrients, or drugs in the body. A biological compound (such as a protein or an antibody) that binds to the substance being evaluated is introduced into a sample of blood or urine. The compound is tagged with radioactivity, and as it links to the target substance, it can easily be found and measured. Because the entire procedure takes place outside the body, no radiation dose is delivered.

- *SPECT (Single Photon Emission Computed Tomography)* is used to evaluate the heart muscle. After the patient exercises, a radioactive substance is introduced into the body. Two sets of pictures, which are taken several hours apart with a gamma camera, produce a three-dimensional image and indicate any blockage. Radiation dose is less than 1 rad.

- *MRI (Magnetic Resonance Imaging)* is used to study tissue, musculo-skeletal problems, and joint diseases including rheumatoid arthritis, osteoarthritis, and tumors within the spinal cord. The patient is placed inside a magnetic coil that has up to 30,000 times the force of the Earth's magnetic field. A computer produces diagnostic images while protons line up in response to the magnet. The protons are then moved out of line by radio-transmitted pulses; they re-form when the transmitter is turned off. No ionizing radiation is produced; however, an electromagnetic field is generated.

- *Ultrasound Imaging, or Sonography* (which produces sonograms) is used to examine the density of soft tissue. It can reveal lumps, tumors, gallstones, and other conditions that require further study. A transducer converts electrical energy into sound waves that bounce off body structures, then go back to the transducer, while an electronic picture of the process is formed. No radioactive material is used and no radiation is delivered.

## WHAT YOU CAN DO ON A PERSONAL LEVEL

If you need a diagnostic x-ray(s), be sure to note the following suggestions.

☐ Before an x-ray is taken, be certain it is necessary for diagnosis or treatment. Even though effective dosage has been lowered for many procedures, such as mammography and dental diagnosis, x-rays should be taken only when absolutely necessary.

☐ Keep a record of all x-rays. Your doctor may be able to use a previous x-ray instead of ordering a new one.

☐ Ask for a copy of your film each time an x-ray is taken. Doctors and medical offices often destroy charts and x-rays after seven years.

☐ If you are pregnant or there is a chance that you might be pregnant, make sure you tell your doctor before any x-rays are taken.

☐ Before an x-ray is taken, make sure the technician is certified and that the equipment has been safety-tested and inspected.

☐ Always use an x-ray shield to protect reproductive organs and other parts of your body that are not being x-rayed.

☐ Discuss all available procedures with your doctor if you need treatment. Find out how much radiation dosage (measured in rads) each procedure delivers. A chest x-ray delivers approximately .05 rads. According to the American College of Radiology, the average American receives .36 rads of radiation each year, over half of it from natural environmental sources.

## HOW TO GET MORE INVOLVED

Education is your strongest defense against unnecessary x-ray procedures. The prudent use of x-rays for diagnosis and treatment, as well as an awareness of alternative diagnostic tools, are the best ways to arm yourself.

☐ For further information on x-rays and diagnostic alternatives, contact:

The American College of Radiology
1891 Preston White Drive
Reston, VA 22091
(703) 648-8900

# LIFESTYLE

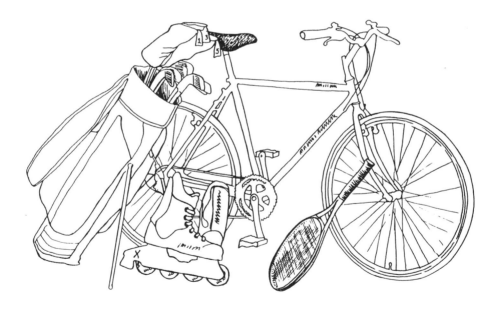

# Chapter 27

# AIDS

More than 1 million people in the United States are infected with the HIV (human immunodeficiency virus) antibody. Carriers of HIV often contract AIDS (acquired immune deficiency syndrome) within a few years of exposure, but infection may precede the onset of symptoms for up to ten years. To date, evidence indicates that all HIV carriers will eventually develop AIDS, although according to June Osborn, M.D., a member of the World Health Organization (WHO) Global Commission on AIDS, some people known to have been infected in 1978 were still well thirteen years later in 1991. The cases of individuals infected with HIV are rising sharply in developing countries. The World Health Organization predicts that in addition to the 10 million people already infected worldwide, there will be another 30 million infected by the year 2000.

HIV, which replicates itself in the white blood cells, is found in and can be transmitted through blood, semen, and vaginal fluids. Other body fluids in which HIV can be found are urine, perspiration, and tears, but there has been no documented evidence proving that HIV can be transmitted through these fluids. Infected fluids must enter the body in order for one to become infected. Infection does not depend on direct access to the bloodstream; certain cells on the surface of mucous membranes that are located on the vaginal and anal walls and in the mouth are also susceptible.

HIV is a fragile virus. According to Dr. Peter Drotman of the Centers for Disease Control (CDC) Division of HIV/AIDS, HIV can be killed with bona fide detergents (but not soaps), alcohol, water that has been heated to 56°C (most hot tap water reaches this temperature), or a solution of one cup of chlorine bleach per gallon of water.

No studies have yet proven that AIDS can be transmitted through the air, through insect bites, by touching objects or surfaces handled by people with the disease, or through casual contact such as shaking hands or hugging. AIDS is not transmitted by dining in restaurants, attending public events, or by socializing with people who have AIDS.

The first documented case that strongly suggests HIV transmission by a health-care professional to a patient occurred when a Stuart, Florida dentist allegedly infected five of his patients before his death in 1989. Also reported are a growing number of health-care workers who have been infected on the job through contact with the blood of patients.

In July of 1991, Dr. Louis W. Sullivan of the United States Department of Health and Human Services, announced a new set of guidelines to all health-care workers. These guidelines, drafted by the CDC, are aimed especially at doctors, dentists, and other health-care workers who are involved with procedures in which blood exposure could cause transmission of HIV. An urgent recommendation for the careful following of the "Universal Precautions" against infection is called for whenever an invasive procedure causing blood-to-blood exposure takes place. These standard procedures include such actions as thorough sterilization of equipment in an autoclave, careful handling and disposing of hypodermic needles and other sharp instruments, the wearing of rubber gloves when appropriate, and any other precaution that may be necessary to prevent blood-to-blood exposure.

You are a high-risk candidate for AIDS if you:

- are an intravenous (IV) drug user.
- are the recipient of a blood transfusion.
- are the recipient of an organ transplant.

- have had an invasive medical procedure performed by an AIDS-infected practitioner.
- have had unprotected sex with multiple partners.
- were born to an AIDS-infected mother.

The AIDS antibody test does not detect the presence of the AIDS virus but measures the presence of HIV antibodies, which form if you have been exposed. Most people develop HIV antibodies three to six months after exposure; on the other hand, it may take up to two years for the antibodies to develop. In order to achieve accurate results if you are sexually active, you should be celibate (or monogamous, if both partners are to be tested) for at least six months before taking the test.

### WHAT YOU CAN DO ON A PERSONAL LEVEL

Guard yourself against AIDS. There are steps you can take to lower your risks.

☐ If you are sexually active, have yourself tested to see if you have been exposed to HIV. If you have had multiple sexual partners, and one of those partners has had sexual contact with someone who carried the virus, you might be infected as well.

☐ The only way to be certain that you will not be exposed to the sexual transmission of AIDS is to be celibate or to have a monogamous sexual relationship with someone who has tested negative for HIV.

☐ Use a condom during sexual relations, but be aware that its use is not a guarantee against AIDS transmission. While widely discussed as a preventive solution, the 1988 Surgeon General's report on AIDS stresses that the use of condoms in sexual relations "offers substantial protection but does not guarantee total protection." Studies show that condoms, though not a solution to the problem, continue to provide the best available protection against the sexual transmission of AIDS.

☐ Make sure your dentist, doctor, and any other health-care professionals follow the "Universal Precautions" provided by the Department of Health and Human Services. These standards call for the proper sterilization of intruments, careful use of and disposal of hypodermic needles and other sharp instruments, the use of rubber gloves when necessary, and any other precaution that may be necessary to prevent blood-to-blood exposure.

☐ For further information on testing, transmission, safe-sex practices, and other issues relating to AIDS, contact:

Gay Men's Health
  Crisis Hotline
(212) 807-6655

U.S.Public Health
  Service
(800) 342-AIDS

Project Inform Hotline
(800) 822-7422
(800) 334-7422 (California)

### HOW TO GET MORE INVOLVED

Take an active stand in the war against AIDS.

☐ Show your concern through support of the following organizations, which are active in AIDS involvement. (Additional information on the organizations is found beginning on page 269.)

Gay Men's Health Crisis
129 West 20th Street
New York, NY 10011
(212) 807-6664

Project Inform
1965 Market Street – Room 220
San Francisco, CA 94103
(800) 822-7422
(800) 334-7422 (California)

National Women's
  Health Network
1325 G Street, NW
Washington, DC 20005
(202) 347-1140

# Chapter 28

# COSMETICS AND PERSONAL-CARE PRODUCTS

Cosmetics have been used since as far back as 3500 B.C., when perfumed hair oils were placed in the tombs of Egyptian kings. Under the 1938 Federal Food, Drug and Cosmetic (FDC) Act, cosmetics are defined as substances that are designed to enhance appearance or promote personal cleansing (soap is exempted and is not regulated). The FDC Act covers all articles that are intended to be "rubbed, poured, sprinkled or sprayed on, introduced into, or otherwise applied to the human body . . . for cleansing, beautifying, promoting attractiveness or altering the appearance of the body without affecting the body's structure or functions."

Formulations that are intended to diagnose, improve or cure a disease or condition, and that affect the body's structure or function, are classified as drugs. (Some dual-function products, such as a deodorant that is also an antiperspirant, are classified as both.)

Registration of cosmetic products and formulas as well as cosmetic testing is voluntary. The FDC Act does require that all cosmetic ingredients, except those considered to be "trade secrets," be listed on product labels.

Most people use no more than fifteen cosmetic products regularly. It is worth taking the time to find out what these products contain.

*Being Beautiful,* published by Ralph Nader's Center for the Study of Responsive Law, lists the most common known and suspected cancer-causing ingredients in cosmetics and personal-care products. Table 28.1 lists these ingredients as well as the products in which they are most commonly found. Of course, not every product listed in Table 28.1 necessarily contains the harmful ingredient listed. Be sure to read product labels carefully.

**Table 28.1   Known and Suspected Cancer-Causing Ingredients in Cosmetics and Personal-Care Products**

| Ingredient | Purpose | Found In |
|---|---|---|
| Acetylanide | Solvent | Nail polish removers. |
| Acetic acid | Solvent | Creams and lotions; hair dyes. |
| BNPD (2-bromo-2-nitropropane-1,3-diol) | Solvent | Nail polish removers; shampoos and conditioners; creams and lotions. |
| Bronopol | Solvent | Creams and lotions; eye makeup. |
| BHA (Butylated hydroxyanisole) | Antioxidant | Lipsticks; shaving creams; soaps. |
| BHT (Butylated hydroxytoluene) | Antioxidant | Creams and lotions; eye makeup; lipsticks; shaving creams; soaps. |
| Coal tar dyes, as: 4-EMPD (4-ethoxy-m-phenylenediamine);4-MMPD (4-methoxy-m-phenylenediamine); 4-MMPD sulfate (4-methoxy-m-phenylenediamine sulfate); 2,4 DA (2,4 daminoanisole); 2,4 DA sulfate (2,4 daminoan- | Oxidating agents | Hair dyes. |

| Ingredient | Purpose | Found In |
|---|---|---|
| isole sulfate); 2-ni-tro-p-phenylene-diamine; 4-amino-2-nitrophenol; 2,4 TDA (2,4-tolue-nediamine); phe-nylenediamine | | |
| Color additives, as: acid blue 9, 74; acid green 5; acid red 1, 18, 27, 73, 87, 88; acid violet 49; acid yellow 11, 73; basic blue 9; ba-sic orange 2; basic violet 1, 3, 10; chro-mium oxide (green); D&C blue 1, 2, 4; D&C red 4, 9, 17, 19, 22; direct black 38, 131; di-rect blue 6; direct brown 1, 31, 95, 154; external blue 1; external D&C red 8, 11, 13; exter-nal yellow 3; FD&C blue 1; FD&C red 1, 2, 4, 40; FD&C violet 1; HC red 6; iron oxide | Coloring agents | Creams and lotions; sham-poos (regular and dandruff) and conditioners; eye makeup; facial cosmetics; hair dyes; lipsticks; mouth-washes; nail polishes; per-fumes, colognes, and after-shave lotions; shaving creams; soaps; toilet tissue; toothpaste. |
| Cresol | Antiseptic, disinfectant | Dandruff shampoos; per-fumes, colognes, and after-shave lotions. |
| Dibutyl phthalate | Plasticizer | Nail polishes. |
| DEA (Diethano-lamine) | Solvent, emulsifier, detergent | Hair dyes; shampoos and con-ditioners. |
| Dimethyl sulfate | Methylating agent | Facial cosmetics; perfumes, co-lognes, and after-shave lotions. |

| Ingredient | Purpose | Found In |
|---|---|---|
| Estrone | Improves skin texture | Creams and lotions; eye makeup. |
| Ethanol | Antibacterial agent, astringent | Toothpaste. |
| Ethyl carbamate | Solvent | Mouthwash. |
| EDTA (Ethylenediamine tetracetic acid) | Solvent; disinfectant | Eyedrops; eye makeup; facial cosmetics; hair dyes; shampoos and conditioners; soaps. |
| Formaldehyde | Disinfectant, germicide, defoamer, preservative | Contraceptive sponges and spermatocides; shampoos (regular and dandruff) and conditioners; deodorants and antiperspirants; eye makeup; feminine hygeine products (deodorants, douches); hair sprays; mouthwash; nail polishes and removers; perfumes, colognes, and after-shave lotions; soaps; toilet tissue; toothpastes. |
| Hydroquinone | Promotes skin depigmentation | Creams and lotions; sun creams and lotions. |
| Lead acetate | Astringent, coloring agent | Hair dyes. |
| Methenamine | Antiseptic | Deodorants and antiperspirants; mouthwash. |
| Methyl methacrylate | Thickener | Nail polishes. |
| Phenol | Disinfectant, antiseptic | Creams and lotions; feminine hygiene products (deodorants, douches); mouthwash; nail polish removers; perfumes, colognes, and after-shave lotions; shaving creams; soaps. |

| Ingredient | Purpose | Found In |
|---|---|---|
| P-hydroxyanisole | Antiseptic | Eye makeup; facial cosmetics; lipstick. |
| Polyethelene | Insulating agent, promotes low moisture absorption | Creams and lotions. |
| Polysorbate 80 | Emulsifier, stabilizer | Creams and lotions; deodorants and antiperspirants; sun creams and lotions. |
| PVP (Polyvinylpyrrolidinone) | Clarifier, softener | Dandruff shampoos; denture cleaners; eye makeup; hair dyes; hair sprays; lipsticks; shampoos (regular and dandruff) and conditioners; toothpaste. |
| Quaternium-15 | Antimicrobial agent | Shampoos and conditioners. |
| Sodium carrageenan | Stabilizer, emulsifier | Creams and lotions; toothpaste. |
| Sodium saccharin | Sweetener | Lipstick; mouthwash; toothpaste. |
| Talc (may contain tremolite, a form of asbestos) | Powdering agent | Body powders; eye makeup; facial cosmetics; feminine hygeine products (deodorants, douches); shaving creams. |
| TEA (Triethanolamine) | Coating agent | Eye makeup; hair dyes; shampoos and conditioners; shaving creams; sun creams and lotions; facial cosmetics. |
| Toluene | Solvent | Nail polish removers. |
| Trichloroethylene | Solvent, degreasing agent | Creams and lotions; perfumes, colognes, and aftershave lotions. |
| Xylene | Solvent | Nail polish removers. |
| Zinc sulfate | Astringent | Shaving creams. |

## WHAT YOU CAN DO ON A PERSONAL LEVEL

The following suggestions can help make nontoxic personal-care products a natural part of your life.

☐ Read labels carefully, and if there is any doubt whatsoever about what the product contains, write to the manufacturer requesting a list of ingredients. If they refuse to name "secret" ingredients, switch products.

☐ Avoid the ingredients that are commonly found in cosmetics and personal-care products (see Table 28.1).

☐ If you find that products you use contain any known or suspected carcinogens, notify the manufacturer that you will switch to another brand. Let the manufacturer know that you will not use their product until the carcinogenic ingredient(s) has been removed.

☐ Buy products with simple formulas without artificial colors. Buy pure, unscented soap. Some old-fashioned products are both pure and inexpensive, such as witch hazel, which is an excellent astringent. Rosewater and glycerin is an effective moisturizing lotion.

☐ A mixture of 1 ½ teaspoons of unflavored gelatin in a cup of warm water has the same effect as mousse when combed through the hair. This gelatin mixture will keep for approximately two weeks unrefrigerated. After two weeks (or if a faintly sour odor is detected), make a new batch of "mousse."

☐ Rinse your mouth with baking soda, salt, or mint tea. Never use a mouthwash with a 25 percent or higher alcohol content. A study by the National Cancer Institute, reported in *Cancer Research* in June 1991, found a potential risk of oral cancer among long-term users of high-alcohol content mouthwashes.

☐ Replace toothpaste with baking soda, talcum powder with corn starch, makeup remover with unscented vegetable jelly (available in natural foods stores), facial scrubs with fuller's earth, expensive moisturizing oils with pure vegetable oils (especially avocado oil), and deodorant with baking soda.

☐ Use products that are unscented. Instead of perfumes and colognes, use essential oils from natural plant sources. Pure oils are labeled "absolute," "concrete," or "true." They should be diluted with vegetable oil (or vodka) before application.

☐ Use products thoughtfully. For instance, rub mousse into towel-dried hair, not into your scalp. Your skin is porous, and all chemicals penetrate it to some extent.

☐ Avoid all spray products, aerosol and non-aerosol. Even though sprays no longer contain chlorofluorocarbons (CFCs), they still contain hydrocarbon compounds. When hydrocarbons combine with oxides of nitrogen in the presence of sunlight, ground-level ozone (a major component of smog) is formed. Polluting compounds may be in the propellant or in the spray itself. Additionally, particles in the spray can remain airborne for several minutes, even in well-ventilated areas. If inhaled, these particles can lodge in the lungs for years, increasing the risk of lung cancer and birth defects. If you must use spray products, hold your breath while spraying, then leave the area immediately and allow the spray to settle.

Pump-spray containers that use normal air, not gas propellants or CFCs, are available for under $10.00 from the following company:

LDSystems, Inc.
Suite 2200
908 South Tryon Street
Charlotte, NC 28202
(704) 332-2336

☐ To find nontoxic cosmetics and personal-care products, check with your local natural foods store, or order directly from:

Aubrey Organics
4419 N. Manhattan Avenue
Tampa, FL 33614
(800) 282-7394

Baudelaire, Inc.
Forest Road
Marlow, NH 03456
(800) 327-2324

*Complete lines of skin-care and hair-care products, makeup, and bath products. Baby products: shampoo, bath soap, and lotions.*

*Body-care products: shampoos, soaps, bath and skin oils, toothpaste. Baby products: powders, bath oils, sun lotions.*

Body Shop
45 Horsehill Road
Cedar Knolls, NJ 07927-2014
(800) 541-2535

*Complete lines of skin- and hair-care products, and makeup. Baby products: creams, lotions, powders, soaps.*

Cernitin America
345 West Leffel Lane
PO Box 1928
Springfield, OH 45501
(800) 831-9505

*Complete lines of skin-care and hair-care products.*

The Chishti Company
PO Box 79
Oxford, NY 13830
(800) 344-7172

*Natural perfume oils.*

Desert Essence Cosmetics
PO Box 588
Topanga, CA 90290
(213) 455-1046

*Complete lines of body-care, hair-care, and mouth-care products.*

Dry Creek Herb Farm
13935 Dry Creek Road
Auburn, CA 95603
(916) 878-2441

*Herbal oils, soaps, bath products.*

Rachel Perry
9111 Mason Avenue
Chatsworth, CA 91311
(800) 624-7001
(818) 888-5881

*Complete lines of skin- and body-care products, and makeup.*

Tom's of Maine
Railroad Avenue
Kennebunk, ME 04043
(207) 985-2944

*Mouth-care products, shaving products, shampoos, deodorants.*

Weleda, Inc.
841 South Main Street
Spring Valley, NY 10977
(914) 356-6145

*Complete lines of skin-care, mouth-care, and bath products; deodorants; massage oils. Baby products: creams, lotions, powders, soaps.*

☐ To order a copy of *Being Beautiful*, a book filled with consumer health and safety advice on skin, nail, eye, and hair products, send a check or money order in the amount of $10.00 (price includes shipping and handling) to:

*Being Beautiful*
Center for the Study of Responsive Law
PO Box 19367
Washington, DC 20036
(202) 387-8030

☐ The following books provide further helpful, healthful information on cosmetics and personal-care products.

*A Consumer's Dictionary of Cosmetic Ingredients* by Ruth Winter. NY: Crown Publishers, 1984.

*Body and Soul* by Anita Roddick. NY: Crown Publishers, 1991.

*The Natural Pharmacy Product Guide* by Richard Israel. Garden City Park, NY: Avery Publishing Group, 1991.

*Natural Skin Care* by Cherie de Haas. Garden City Park, NY: Avery Publishing Group, 1987.

## HOW TO GET MORE INVOLVED

Speak out on issues concerning harmful ingredients in cosmetics and personal-care products.

☐ To send the strongest message possible, use your economic power to affect change. Write to manufacturers and let them know that you will not buy their products until harmful ingredients are removed. Your voice will be heard loud and clear.

☐ Write a letter to the Food and Drug Administration (FDA). Express your concerns and urge the FDA to implement stricter controls on the harmful additives used in cosmetics and personal-care products. Encourage the FDA to require all ingredients (including those that are considered "trade secrets") to be listed on product labels.

Consumer Affairs
Food and Drug Administration
5600 Fishers Lane – HFE 88
Rockville, MD 20857

# Chapter 29

# ESTROGEN AND BIRTH CONTROL PILLS

Millions of American women take estrogen, either in the form of birth control pills or as hormone-replacement therapy after menopause. The United States Department of Health publication *Cancer Prevention: Good News, Better News, Best News* points out that women who have taken large doses of estrogen for menopause symptoms have an increased risk of cancer of the endometrium, the lining of the uterus.

The risk of estrogen-related uterine cancer increases proportionately with high dosages and with long duration of use. Animals that have been given estrogen for long periods of time have developed cancers of the cervix, vagina, uterus, and liver. Additionally, the Centers for Disease Control (CDC) reports that there is a direct link between the use of menopausal estrogen and an increased risk of breast cancer. This risk is especially high in women with fibrocystic breast disease (benign breast tumors) or cervical dysplasia (cervical abnormality). Many breast cancers are estrogen response (ER) positive, which means that they need estrogen to grow.

A 1989 report of studies conducted by the Boston University School of Medicine, the Food and Drug Administration (FDA); the Uniformed Services University of the Health Sciences at Bethesda, Maryland; and England's Royal College of General Practitioners, Manchester Research Unit also reveals that some birth control pill users have a higher risk of cervical and breast cancer, especially if they have a close relative with one of these cancer types. The Boston University study also indicated that women under the age of forty-five may double their breast-cancer risk by taking birth control pills.

In 1990, the *Journal of the National Cancer Institute* reported that Swedish studies found a 1 to 1½ times higher breast-cancer risk for long-term users of estrogen-replacement therapy, and a nearly 6 times higher risk for premenopausal women who began using the pill in their teenage years.

In other studies, birth control pills have been shown to actually diminish the risk of uterine and ovarian cancers (and in September 1991, the *New England Journal of Medicine* reported that estrogen-replacement therapy may reduce the risk of heart disease in menopausal women). These cancers, however, are far less common than breast cancer, which afflicts one of every nine women in the United States.

## WHAT YOU CAN DO ON A PERSONAL LEVEL

If you presently take or plan to take birth control pills or estrogen-replacement therapy, consider the following suggestions.

☐ In light of recent concerns about the birth control pill's link to breast cancer, the National Women's Health Network advises that women should not use the pill for longer than three years. Then they should switch to an alternative form of contraception.

☐ Do not take oral contraceptives or estrogen-replacement therapy drugs if you have relatives with breast cancer, especially a mother or sister. Ask your doctor or your local Planned Parenthood agency for information on alternative contraceptive methods.

☐ Examine your breasts every month. Information on breast self-examination is available from the American Cancer Society (see the white pages of your telephone book for your local chapter) or from the National Cancer Institute Hotline (800-4-CANCER).

☐  Ask your doctor when you should have a baseline mammogram, how to schedule regular follow-up care, and how to begin an exercise program if you are not presently exercising. Exercise tends to lower estrogen levels in some women. Make sure you have a Pap test every six to twelve months.

☐  Women have reportedly relieved symptoms of menopause, such as hot flashes and leg cramps, by taking vitamin E, starting with 130 mg (200 IU) daily and increasing the dosage by 130 mg (200 IU) every two weeks until they are taking 500 to 800 mg (800–1200 IU) daily.

☐  If you are menopausal, include plenty of soybeans, peas, and other legumes in your diet. Legumes are rich sources of natural female hormones (estrogen).

☐  To prevent osteoporosis, take vitamin B₆, extra vitamin C, and 1200–1500 mg of calcium daily. Calcium is better absorbed and retained in the bones in later years if supplementation is begun by the age of thirty. Calcium retention is also enhanced by weight-bearing exercise, such as walking, jogging, rebounding (jumping on a trampoline), and tennis.

☐  For several thousand years, Chinese women have used the herb anjelica *(Anjelica archangelica)* to prevent hot flashes during menopause. Two capsules are taken three times a day until symptoms disappear, then one capsule is taken daily until the menopause stage is over. Other herbs used for relief of symptoms of menopause are passion flower, black cohosh, damiana, licorice (not to be taken by those with high blood pressure), raspberry, sage, and dong quai.

## HOW TO GET MORE INVOLVED

To get actively involved in the area of women's health issues, try the following.

☐  Support consumer-oriented groups and agencies that focus on women's health issues. (Additional information on the organizations is found beginning on page 269.)

National Women's
  Health Network
1325 G Street, NW
Washington, DC 20005
(202) 347-1140

Public Citizen Health
  Research Group
2000 P Street, NW
Washington, DC 20036
(202) 833-3000

# Chapter 30

# LACK OF EXERCISE

The link between exercise and cancer has been researched for well over seventy-five years. As early as 1911, James Ewing, a leading cancer researcher, noted that he saw the highest occurrence of malignancy among people who were physically inactive. He observed that cancer was more prevalent among the "well-to-do and indolent" than among the "poor and (physically) overworked."

Further research continued to connect a lack of exercise to cancer. In a 1962 study led by Drs. S.A. Hoffman and K.E. Paschkis, malignancies were completely reversed in cancer-prone mice after they were injected with an extract from the fatigued muscle tissue of mice who had just exercised to the point of exhaustion.

A 1981 UCLA study concluded that a mere five minutes of exercise increased the production of natural killer blood cells. A 1985 study that was conducted at the Harvard School of Public Health examined 2,622 women between the ages of twenty-one and eighty (approximately half of whom had been college athletes). The study concluded that women who were active in athletics during their college years had lower lifetime rates of cancer of the reproductive system (ovarian, uterine, cervical, and vaginal) and of the breasts than non-athletes. In addition, research reported at the 1991 meeting of the American Institute for Cancer Research concluded that regular exercise reduced risks of both colon cancer and cardiovascular disease in an ongoing study of 57,000 college graduates.

These results may relate to the fact that exercise tends to lower estrogen levels. High estrogen levels are parallel to elevated risks of breast and reproductive system cancers. Aerobic exercise also helps maintain a beneficial ratio of high density lipoproteins (HDLs) to low density lipoproteins (LDLs), which can enhance immune system function. LDLs are sometimes referred to as the bad cholesterol because they deposit plaque on the arterial walls. HDLs are referred to as the good cholesterol because they carry this artery-clogging plaque from arterial walls to the liver for processing and elimination.

In June 1990, the *Journal of the National Cancer Institute* reported that colon and rectal cancer risk was elevated among men employed in sedentary professions. Studies at the University of Southern California School of Medicine and at the Department of Social and Preventive Medicine, State University of New York at Buffalo also found a greater risk of colon cancer in men whose jobs did not keep them physically active.

Dr. Hans Selye and other researchers believe that exercise might reduce cancer incidence by appropriately channeling stress. O. Carl Simonton, M.D., who, in the 1970s, pioneered the use of visual imagery in the treatment of cancer, observed that some of his most successful patients were those who followed a regular, vigorous exercise program. Dr. Simonton also believes that people who are committed to regular exercise tend to develop a healthier physiological profile, which correlates with improved prognosis.

Aerobic exercise increases the body's need for oxygen; a high level of oxygen in the blood can have a negative effect on cancer cells. Nobel Prize winning biochemist Otto Heinrich Warburg, M.D., notes that lack of oxygen can cause cellular damage that leads to cancer, but regular exercise provides oxygen to cells that can help protect them. As the blood vessels expand to deliver more oxygenated blood, the increased blood flow delivers more of the immune system's protective blood cells and healthful hormones to all parts of the body.

In addition to relieving tension, exercise also speeds up the metabolic processes, including elimination of toxins through the liver, skin, kidneys, and colon. After exercising, the body's metabolism can continue to be affected for up to fifteen hours. Exercise can also help prevent obesity by burning excess calories and/or by suppressing the appetite.

## WHAT YOU CAN DO ON A PERSONAL LEVEL

Reduce your risks of certain cancers through exercise.

□ *If you do not currently exercise, be sure to check with your doctor or health-care provider before getting involved in any type of exercise program.*

□ Exercise aerobically for thirty minutes at least three times a week. Gradually work up to forty to sixty minutes, five times a week. Brisk walking, rebounding (jumping on a mini-trampoline), dancing, swimming, cycling, tennis, racquetball, skipping rope, rowing, cross-country skiing, roller skating, and stair climbing are good aerobic exercises. Running is not recommended because the impact of each stride is approximately four times the body's weight. This impact creates an enormous amount of stress on the knees and the skeletal system, especially on the joints and tendons. Start to build your endurance slowly, with a comfortable activity such as walking or stationary bicycling with low resistance.

□ Consider joining a general conditioning exercise class or health/fitness club.

□ Additional information on exercise and good health is found in the following books.

*The Aerobics Program for Total Well-Being* by Kenneth Cooper. NY: M. Evans & Co., 1982.

*Cancer and Nutrition: A Ten Point Plan to Reduce Your Chances of Getting Cancer* by Charles B. Simone, M.D. Garden City Park, NY: Avery Publishing Group, 1992.

*Jumping for Health* by Dr. Morton Walker. Garden City Park, NY: Avery Publishing Group, 1982.

*The Stress of Life* by Hans Selye. NY: McGraw Hill, 1956.

## HOW TO GET MORE INVOLVED

It is critical for exercise to be given a high priority in our lives; the documented physical and mental health benefits are too important to ignore. One way that you can spread the word and encourage others to become more physically fit is through your own visible, active involvement.

☐ Join a local organized sports league. No matter what age you are, there is always a sport that you can join. Most neighborhoods offer softball, tennis, swimming, basketball, soccer, and bowling leagues. Choose something that suits your interest and ability. Contact local parks departments, town halls, police departments, churches, sporting goods stores, and libraries for information on sports activities that are available in your area.

☐ Help organize a bike-a-thon or walk-a-thon for a charitable cause. Encourage your church, school, or a local business organization to sponsor such an event.

☐ If you are in good general health, consider joining a bicycling or a rowing club. These groups often sponsor marathons and other activities. Check with your state's Department of Recreation for names and contacts of local organizations.

☐ Contact the President's Council on Physical Fitness and Sports. Sponsored by the United States Public Health Service, the Council's goal is to keep Americans (children and adults) healthy through exercise. Through its awards-incentive program, individuals can choose from among fifty-one activities. For additional information, contact:

President's Council on Physical Fitness and Sports
Washington, DC 20001
(202) 272-3421

# Chapter 31

# OBESITY

There is a direct correlation between low-calorie intake and reduced cancer rates. Obesity, defined as being 10 percent over ideal body weight, is a risk factor for many diseases, including cancer.

A twelve-year study involving over 750,000 people was conducted by the American Cancer Society. This study concluded that overweight people are at a greater risk for uterine, kidney, and stomach cancers. Particularly high are the risks of cancers of the endometrium, gallbladder, cervix, colon, rectum, and breast. The study found that the more overweight the person, the greater the cancer risk.

The American Cancer Society has warned that obesity is associated with a 55 percent higher cancer risk for women and a 33 percent higher risk for men. In particular, a 1991 report of studies that were conducted at the University of South Florida at Tampa linked upper-body fat (above the hips) in women to higher rates of cancers of the breast and the uterine lining. Women with a high waist-to-hip ratio of body fat have high levels of circulating estrogen, which may be a factor in the growth and development of some hormonally promoted tumors. Low body weight is related to better health in general as well as to lower cancer rates.

## WHAT YOU CAN DO ON A PERSONAL LEVEL

The following suggestions can help lower your risks of health-related problems due to obesity.

☐ Eat less. Eat smaller portions. As children, we needed and consumed much more food per pound of body weight than we need as adults. It is important for us, as adults, to make a conscious calorie reduction in our diets.

☐ There is a higher incidence of cancer among those whose bodies tend to be apple-shaped. If you carry your body weight in this android pattern (around and above the waist), adopt a long-term weight-reduction plan. Commit yourself to maintaining your weight loss. Losing even 5 percent of your overall weight can be beneficial to your health.

☐ Set a reasonable and attainable weight goal based on your body type, family history, and on your ability to exercise and regulate your eating. Whatever your weight goal, focus on maintaining your weight loss. Fluctuating weight can cause hypertension and can increase your risk of heart disease.

☐ Cut out processed foods and eat more complex carbohydrates and fiber. Do not eat simple carbohydrates in refined sugars and grain products because they provide no nutritional benefits. As we become adults, our metabolism slows and we need less food. It is imperative that the foods we consume provide our full nutritional requirements for good health.

☐ Chew each mouthful of food until it becomes liquid. Well-chewed food is absorbed more rapidly in the intestines, and it provides a feeling of fullness. Because food that has been well-chewed passes through the intestinal tract more quickly, there is less time for chemicals that may be present to promote or initiate cellular changes that can lead to cancer. Also, as well-chewed food is absorbed, the blood sugar level rises and suppresses the appetite.

☐ Exercise regularly. Calories continue to burn after the exercise period is over. Exercise helps lower the "setpoint," which is the body's natural or currently maintained weight.

# Aspartame

*The sugar substitute aspartame is made from aspartic acid and phenylalinine, which break down into amino acids (building blocks of protein) in the body. Reports of dizziness, headaches, epileptic-like seizures, and menstrual problems have resulted after aspartame ingestion. Often the symptoms are very much like those of MSG sensitivity, or "Chinese restaurant syndrome."*

*An early aspartame study on rats showed an increase of brain tumors, but a second study on a different strain of rats did not find the same elevated risk. Consumer-protection organizations such as Center for Science in the Public Interest continue to urge the FDA to require aspartame's manufacturer to conduct a definitive study.*

*Large doses of phenylalanine can cause seizures in people with a particular disorder called* phynylketonuria. *Phenylketonuria is a birth defect in which an enzyme needed to change the amino acid phenylalanine into another substance is missing. Buildup of phenylalanine is poisonous to brain tissue. This defect occurs in one of every 20,000 newborns. In these infants, ingestion of phenylalanine could result in mental retardation.*

☐ Do not eat for at least three and preferably four hours before going to bed. The body does not burn calories efficiently during periods of sleep.

☐ Do not use sugar substitutes, which might increase your cravings for sugar. Saccharin is also a known carcinogen, and aspartame (marketed as Equal or NutraSweet) may cause altered brain function and behavioral changes ( inset above).

☐ Be aware that protein and carbohydrates provide four calories per gram, fat provides nine, and alcohol provides seven. A

1988 study at the Stanford Center for Research in Disease Prevention concluded that fat calories count more (cause more weight gain) than calories from complex carbohydrates, because they are burned less efficiently. This means that the same number of calories that help maintain normal weight when consumed as complex carbohydrates may cause obesity when they are consumed as fat.

☐ Eat plenty of vegetables, fruits, legumes, and grains, which are low in calories and fat, high in fiber, and give a feeling of fullness.

☐ If you need help returning to and maintaining your ideal weight, consider a support program that encourage weight-reduction through healthy lifestyle changes (not fad diets). Check local yellow pages under *Weight Control Services*.

☐ Hypnosis and self-hypnosis techniques have been effective in treating people who are chronically obese and unable to lose weight.

☐ For additional information, see the chapters on *Dietary Fat*, *Dietary Imbalance*, and *Lack of Exercise*.

## HOW TO GET MORE INVOLVED

Take an active stand on nutrition and health.

☐ Support organizations that keep the public informed of nutritional breakthroughs and other weight-control information. (Additional information on the organizations is found beginning on page 269.)

Center for Science in the
  Public Interest
Suite 300
1875 Connecticut Avenue, NW
Washington, DC 20009-5728
(202) 332-9110

Community Nutrition
  Institute
Suite 500
2001 S Street, NW
Washington, DC 20009
(202) 462-4700

Public Citizen
2000 P Street, NW
Washington, DC 20036
(202) 833-3000

# Chapter 32

# SILICONE IMPLANTS

According to the United States Food and Drug Administration (FDA), approximately 2 million women in the United States have had breast implants. These implants have been used since 1964 for both cosmetic and reconstructive purposes; about 20 percent of these women have had implant surgery to reconstruct breasts following mastectomies. Prior to 1992, most implants were filled with silicone (a gel-like combination of silicon, oxygen, and hydrocarbons).

The law giving the FDA the authority to regulate medical devices such as implants was passed in 1976. This law grandfathered devices already on the market, including breast implants, because products already in use were presumed to be safe. However, if questions about a grandfathered device arise over time, the FDA has the authority to require the manufacturer to prove that its product is safe and effective. In 1991, in response to studies that linked silicone implants to cancer, the FDA exercised this authority with manufacturers of breast implants. In January 1992, after reviewing manufacturers' evidence, FDA Commissioner David A. Kessler announced a moratorium on silicone implants while the FDA reviewed whether the public health need for the devices outweighed new information on implant risk.

In April 1992, the FDA panel announced its decision. Women seeking silicone gel implants following a mastectomy will be able to get them, as well as women who require reconstruction resulting from breast disease or a severe congenital breast deformity. Women who want silicone gel implants for cosmetic augmentation will have a much more difficult time. (Saline implants remain on the market.)

All of the women receiving the implants are to be part of closely controlled, three-year clinical trials. These trials have been established to focus on the safety issues surrounding the silicone implants, including how much they leak or harden, how often they rupture, and whether they cause autoimmune disorders.

The FDA has outlined the following three-stage breast implant program:

1. *Stage one.* Silicone gel implants are available immediately for those women who are presently ready for reconstructive surgery, and for those women whose existing implants have ruptured.

2. *Stage two.* By mid-1992, implant recipients will include women seeking reconstruction due to cancer, breast disease, or severe congenital deformity.

3. *Stage three.* This last group will include a small group of women desiring cosmetic breast augmentation.

Silicone breast implants may pose a cancer risk specifically and directly to the breast, and/or to distant parts of the body. One breast-related risk is that mammograms of breasts with implants are less likely to detect the presence of a tumor at its smallest, most treatable stage. In some cases, fibrous tissue grows around the implant, causing discomfort, pain, and hardening of the breast. Another concern is that the implant's outer envelope may rupture, releasing its gel filling.

The most common breast-related risk is *capsular contracture,* which can occur either immediately after surgery or many years later. Capsular contracture results from the shrinkage of the layer of scar tissue that forms around any implanted object. As the scar tissue shrinks, the breasts can become hard, lumpy, painful, uneven, and deformed. If the problem is severe, a *closed compression capsulotomy* may be recommended. In this procedure, pressure is applied to the breast in order to break up the hardening tissue. However, the pressure itself can cause bleeding or a rupturing of the implant. If bleeding or rupture occur, the patient may require further surgery to remove scar tissue or to have entire implants removed.

Risks to distant parts of the body from silicone breast implants are often more difficult to observe and measure. Even if the implant's outer envelope does not rupture, minute amounts of gel can escape and migrate throughout the body. There is evidence that silicone seepage can enter the lymph nodes and impair a woman's immune system. This impairment causes susceptibility to disorders such as rheumatoid arthritis, scleroderma, or lupus (systemic lupus erythematosus)—a disease of the body's connective tissue.

The greatest concern of most silicone breast implant recipients is their elevated risk of developing cancer. A 1988 study conducted by Dow Corning, a former implant manufacturer, linked silicone gel implants in rats to increased rates of sarcoma. Other studies have shown that the polyurethane-foam coating of implants made by the Bristol-Myers Squibb subsidiary Surgitek—which are sold under the labels Meme and Replicon—may dissolve in the body. As this coating dissolves, it produces a chemical known as TDA (2-toluene diamine), which has been shown to cause cancer of the liver in rats and other research animals.

In the first Federal Court decision to link breast implants to breast cancer, a jury in the United States District Court in New York City concluded that the chemical TDA promoted breast cancer in a woman fifteen months after her painful cosmetic implants were removed. (The foam-coated silicone had been implanted for a total of twenty-two days.) TDA has also been found in the milk of a nursing mother and in the urine of a woman after the removal of her foam-coated implants, which had been in place for seven months. In December 1991, a jury awarded $7.3 million to a California woman with an autoimmune disease, saying that the manufacturer fraudulently failed to disclose the risks of silicone implants.

There are five major types of breast implants. All of them use a silicone rubber balloon, but each has a different outer surface and a different filling.

- *Silicone gel implants* have a smooth outer surface and are filled with a silicone, jello-like gel.

- *Saline implants* have a smooth outer shell and are filled with a saline (salt water) solution. If a saline-filled implant leaks, the salt water is absorbed by the body. The breast will deflate, however, and the implant must be replaced.

- *Double-lumen implants* have a smooth outer surface. They contain a balloon within a balloon. One balloon is filled with silicone gel and the other is filled with water, so that the breast does not deflate completely if there is a leak.

- *Textured implants* have fuzzy outer surfaces of either textured silicone or textured polyurethane sponge that encase the silicone gel. These implants allow the body tissue to grow into them, reducing the risk of capsular contracture.

- *Translucent gel implants* have a textured outer surface and are filled with a water-soluble gel; in the event of a rupture, the gel is eliminated through the kidneys in about four days.

Instead of implants, breasts can also be reconstructed using flap techniques. A woman's own body tissues, usually taken from the abdomen or thighs, is used to build up breasts.

Reconstructed breasts are harder and firmer than natural breasts, and they do not flatten as natural breasts do when a woman lies down. If one breast is reconstructed, the other will usually need to be surgically lifted so that both breasts look similar, but an implanted breast never exactly matches a natural breast. Because reconstructed breasts tend to be flat across the front, some women who have had implants use additional padding in their clothing to achieve a natural look.

## WHAT YOU CAN DO ON A PERSONAL LEVEL

If you have had or are planning to have breast implants, consider the following.

☐ Before having a breast implant, be sure to ask your doctor whether the cosmetic benefits of breast reconstruction outweigh the risks to your health.

☐ If you qualify for a breast implant, strongly consider choosing the saline type. In the event of leakage, saline implants pose the least amount of health risk to the body.

☐ If you have had or are going to have a silicone breast implant, make sure you obtain the brand name of the implant, the name and address of the manufacturer, the model name and number, the lot number, and the model year. The model year is important because many implants manufactured between 1975 and 1985 used thinner bags to hold the silicone gel, and these bags may be more prone to rupture or leakage. Get a copy of the package enclosure that comes with the device. This information should also be in your medical records, because your surgeon will need it if you ever have a problem with your implant.

☐ If you have a breast implant, perform a breast self-exam every month, and have an exam by your physician every six months. Some symptoms of implant leakage or rupture are lumps in the chest, abdomen, or arms; a difference in shape, texture, or appearance in your two breasts; chest pain or burning; stiffness in the chest, shoulder, or upper arm; and lumps under the arms, or enlargement of lymph nodes in the underarm area.

☐ If you have a polyurethane foam-coated implant, be aware that after the device is implanted, the foam will remain intact for about a week. Then, as the implant begins to bond to the breast tissue, the foam will begin to break down, and it should not be disturbed for approximately eighteen months. If a surgeon tries to remove an implant while the foam is breaking down, there is a good chance that foam pieces may separate. Pieces that are left in the breast may become infected.

☐ The risk of removing a breast implant may outweigh the risk of keeping it in place. There is danger of disfiguration, chronic infection, and skin ulceration in the removal of any breast implant.

☐ If you decide to have an implant removed, contact a surgeon who specializes in breast disease. Once removed, check the implant's serial number. Keep the implant in your own possession; it may be useful in planning later treatment or in possible litigation.

☐ If you have a problem with an existing silicone implant, contact the following organization, which works with doctors and researchers who are studying the problems of silicone breast implants. They can advise you on how to proceed with remediation.

Command Trust Implant Information Network
256 South Linden Drive
Beverly Hills, CA 90212
(213) 556-1738

☐ A breast-implant hotline has recently been set up by the Breast Cancer Center of the Albert Einstein Medical Center in Philadelphia, Pennsylvania. This hotline is staffed by a team of nurses who are equipped to answer your questions and concerns on the subject of breast implants.

Einstein Direct
(215) 456-7000

HOW TO GET MORE INVOLVED

Voice your concerns about women's health and safety issues.

☐ Write to officials of the FDA. Urge them to promote stricter testing and controls on silicone products.

Consumer Affairs
Food and Drug Administration
5600 Fishers Lane – HFE 88
Rockville, MD 20857

☐ Support the following organizations, which provide information on and advocate better federal health policies for women. (Additional information on the organizations is found beginning on page 269.)

National Alliance of Breast
  Cancer Organizations
1180 Avenue of the Americas
New York, NY 10036
(212) 719-0154

Public Citizen Health
  Research Group
2000 P Street, NW
Washington, DC 20036
(202) 833-3000

National Women's Health
  Network
1325 G Street, NW
Washington, DC 20005
(202) 347-1140

Y-ME
18220 Harwood Avenue
Chicago, IL
(800) 221-2141 (9–5)
(708) 799-8228 (24 hour)

# Chapter 33

# SMOKING: ACTIVE AND PASSIVE

According to the *Merck Manual*, a widely respected medical reference, smoking causes 90 percent of all lung cancers among men and 70 percent among women. The cancer death rate for male cigarette smokers is more than double that of nonsmokers, and 67 percent higher for female smokers. Additionally, over 53,000 nonsmokers die from environmental tobacco smoke each year. All in all, smoking causes nearly 400,000 deaths annually in the United States, and approximately 2.5 million worldwide, according to the World Health Organization (WHO). In August 1991, the *Journal of the National Cancer Institute* reported that between 1959 and 1982, the risk of lung-cancer death doubled for male cigarettes smokers, and quadrupled for female smokers.

Smoking is also implicated in cancers of the bladder, breast, cervix, colon, esophagus, larynx, kidney, mouth, pancreas, and pharynx, as well as in heart disease, emphysema, and even facial wrinkles. It can make other chemicals more potent; when combined with these chemicals, tobacco's effects are magnified. Smokers exposed to asbestos might increase their cancer risk by 9,000 percent.

Tobacco smoke contains hundreds of chemical substances in the form of gases (including ammonia, aldehydes, carbon monoxide, hydrazine, nitrosamines, and vinyl chloride) and particulates (including polycyclic aromatic hydrocarbons and aromatic amines). Many of these substances cause cancer. According to Barbara Phillips, M.D., of the University of Kentucky Medical Center in Lexington, at least one substance, nicotine, can reduce immune-system function by depressing the activity of natural killer cells.

At least two-thirds of the toxins in tobacco smoke are released from the burning end of cigarettes, cigars, and pipes. These toxins are carried on air currents into the surrounding air. Nearby nonsmokers involuntarily inhale these toxins, breathing in both the unfiltered, burning-end smoke and the smoker's exhaled smoke. In the 1986 Surgeon General's report *The Health Consequences of Involuntary Smoking*, Dr. C. Everett Koop characterized passive (sidestream) smoke as even more hazardous than primary (mainstream) smoke.

A 1990 Environmental Protection Agency (EPA) draft report concluded that in the United States, passive smoke kills 53,000 non-smokers a year. The National Institute for Occupational Safety and Health (NIOSH) estimates that living with a smoker increases a person's risk of contracting cancer by 30 percent. A study reported in the January 1992 edition of *Cancer Epidemiology, Biomarkers & Prevention* found the same 30 percent increase in cancer risk among lifelong nonsmokers when they were exposed to passive smoke at home, at work, and in social settings.

Children of smokers are twice as likely to be in poor health as the children of nonsmokers. Studies conducted in 1991 at Carleton University in Ottawa, Canada, found that even fetuses are affected by tobacco smoke. The Carleton studies concluded that children who were exposed to secondhand, passive smoke and/or whose mothers smoked during the critical nine pre-natal months scored significantly lower on academic tests as well as tests on perception, language, speech, and motor skills. These children also had more behavioral problems. A 1991 study conducted at the University of North Carolina revealed that parental smoking lowered children's cognitive performance test scores significantly, particularly in later years (at the ten-year examination).

Separating smokers and nonsmokers in the same room or area, such as in designated areas of airports, airplanes, and restaurants, reduces exposure to tobacco smoke but does not eliminate it. It is unhealthy to be in any room or space, even a large one, where tobacco is being smoked.

In studies conducted in 1985 and 1988 by the National Institute of Environmental Health Sciences in Research Park, North Carolina, researchers found that overall cancer rates are increasing among children whose parents smoke. The effects of passive smoke accumulate over a lifetime, possibly leading to a four times greater cancer risk, as well as to an increased death rate from heart disease.

Pipe and cigar smokers who do not inhale might reduce their risk of lung cancer, but they increase their risk of oral cancer by holding smoke in their mouths. Cigar and pipe smoke may be even more hazardous to nonsmokers than cigarette smoke, because pipes and cigars produce higher levels of benzo-a-pyrene and other carcinogens. The smoke from one cigar pollutes the air as much as the smoke from four to five cigarettes.

The American Cancer Society points out that there has been a recent resurgence in the use of smokeless tobacco—plug, leaf and snuff. Snuff is tobacco that has been processed into a coarse, moist powder. Snuff is placed between the cheek and gum, so that nicotine and a number of other carcinogens are absorbed through the mucous membrane tissue of the mouth. Users can absorb twice as much nicotine from smokeless tobacco as from cigarettes. Long-time snuff users increase their risk of cheek and gum cancer by 5,000 percent. In 1988, a University of California dental team discovered that nearly half of 1,109 professional baseball players who regularly used snuff or chewing tobacco had oral lesions. In some cases, the lesions disappeared when the players stopped using the snuff and chewing tobacco.

Addiction to nicotine can be stronger than an addiction to any other legal or illegal drug. Former Surgeon General Dr. C. Everett Koop described tobacco smoking as far more costly and deadly than heroin, cocaine, or alcohol.

## WHAT YOU CAN DO ON A PERSONAL LEVEL

Recovering from an addiction is always difficult. The following suggestions may help you quit smoking.

☐ In 1990, Surgeon General Antonia Novello noted that giving up smoking has "major and immediate health benefits," which include lowering cancer risk. Former smokers live longer than continuing smokers. Someone who quits smoking before age fifty has half the risk of dying within the next fifteen years from a smoking-related illness as the continuing smoker does.

☐ In addition to self-determination, the help of medical aids such as gum that contains nicotine, nicotine patches, and/or the help of social support groups, hypnotherapists, psycho-therapists, or counselors may be required. In the final analysis, virtually any system that has successfully helped someone stop smoking may be worth trying.

☐ The Damon and Grace Corporation successfully pioneered group hypnosis for habit control twenty-two years ago. With an 86–87 percent success rate per session, Damon and Grace stop-smoking seminars are conducted nationwide. For a schedule of when the seminar will be conducted in your area, contact:

Damon and Grace Corporation
PO Box 674
Okemos, MI 48805-0674
(800) 4-HABITS

☐ SmokeEnders conducts stop-smoking programs at YM and YWCAs, community centers, and clinics across the country. For more information, contact:

SmokeEnders
37 North 3rd Street
Easton, PA 18047
(215) 250-0700

☐ Stop-smoking programs are also offered through:

American Health
  Foundation
1 Dana Road
Valhalla, NY 10595
(914) 592-2600

American Cancer Society
1599 Clifton Road, NE
Atlanta, GA 30329
(404) 320-3333

☐ An herbal stop-smoking kit is available from:

Dry Creek Herb Farm
1395 Dry Creek Road
Auburn, CA 95603
(916) 878-2441

## HOW TO GET MORE INVOLVED

If you are interested in becoming active in anti-smoking issues, consider the following.

☐ Support the groups and organizations that are active in their fight against smoking. (Additional information on the organizations is found beginning on page 269.)

Action on Smoking
  and Health
2013 H Street, NW
Washington, DC 20006
(202) 659-4310

Group Against Smoking
  Pollution
25 Deaconess Street
Boston, MA 02115
(617) 266-2088

American Lung Association
1740 Broadway
New York, NY 10019
(212) 315-8700

National Women's
  Health Network
1325 G Street, NW
Washington, DC 20005
(202) 347-1140

Americans for Nonsmokers
  Rights
2530 San Pablo Place – Suite J
Berkeley, CA 94702
(415) 841-3032

Smoking Policy Institute
PO Box 20271
Seattle, WA 98102
(206) 324-4444

# Chapter 34

# STRESS

Stress is our physical and emotional response to life's events. Positive experiences, such as winning a competition or attending a happy family reunion, can produce positive stress. Negative experiences, such as the death of a loved one or a chronic illness, often produce negative stress. Stress and our reaction to it affect the entire body, and can play a role in deactivating the body's natural defense system, the immune system.

Most people remain healthy when exposed to cancer-causing substances. However, when the immune system is suppressed, cancer cells that are normally held in check or destroyed—and each of us has cancer cells present in our bodies from time to time—are, instead, able to grow unchecked and multiply.

Until the 1880s, standard medical texts referred to the fact that emotional states affect physical health. From that time until the 1980s, most medical literature ceased to acknowledge this link. However, based on observation and experience, generations of doctors and patients continued to believe that emotions—including those that generate prolonged, unremitting stress—can produce a direct, measurable effect on the body.

The question of exactly how negative stress undermines immunity has been discussed since the days of Galen (140 A.D.) and Plato, but only recently has it begun to be scientifically understood.

In the 1980s, the study of *psychoneuroimmunology,* a relatively new field in which the findings of psychology and immunology are understood as interrelated, began to reveal some of the precise ways in which the mind and emotions influence the body. These findings showed how our emotional states may work to prevent, promote, or change the course of cancer.

One method that links our mind and body—our emotions and immune system—is indirect. The limbic brain (a component of the sub-cortex, or lower, non-intellectual brain) registers and records emotional states and feelings. This recorded information is communicated to the endocrine system through the hypothalamus, which transmits it to the pituitary gland. Hormones that are directly appropriate to the specific negative or positive feelings registered are then released to all parts of the body. These hormones affect the body in a sustained and prolonged way.

Negative or unexpressed feelings, such as sadness, despair, worry, fear, anger, grief, hostility, frustration, helplessness, and hopelessness, release hormones that can block or weaken the immune system's defense mechanisms. Conversely, positive feelings of hope, joy, faith, love, excitement, safety, protection, comfort, pleasure, trust, peace, harmony, and fulfillment generate hormones that strengthen and enhance the immune system, including its ability to prevent cancer.

Some negative feelings are unavoidable and are, in fact, appropriate responses to life's events. Dismissing or repressing these negative feelings can prolong their ill effects. For example, a healthy response to sadness and grief that has been caused by the death of a loved one usually involves experiencing these painful negative feelings acutely at first. As time passes, the intensity diminishes until the painful feelings are resolved or integrated into the totality of the life experience.

Stress also affects us through another direct mind-body link, from the nervous system to the immune system. The limbic brain transmits messages prompted by specific positive or negative feelings to a neuroreceptor located on each white blood cell. White blood cells respond with behavior that is appropriate to the specific recorded feelings: they either support or undermine the immune system's healthy functions.

Stress can also activate the "fight-or-flight" response, causing *catecholamines*—adrenalin (epinephrine) and noradrenalin (norepinephrine)—cortisol, and other hormones to be released. A surge of adrenalin can enable one to flee in response to a perceived threat, or to fight it aggressively, sometimes with seemingly superhuman strength. When our forefathers faced killer animals in the wild or warriors on the battlefield, this adrenalin surge gave them the power to resolve the problem by following their lifesaving instincts. In today's generally less primitive circumstances, however, there isn't always an opportunity to resolve stress. For instance, when a company lays off an employee, he usually does not run for his life, and he seldom murders his former boss.

When the activated fight-or-flight response isn't followed by stress-resolving behavior, hormones continue to be released that, over time, depress the immune system. Cortisol, in particular, can reduce the number and inhibit the performance of beneficial T-lymphocytes (T-cells), T-helpers, and other natural killer cells.

*Advances: The Journal of Mind-Body Health* reported in 1991 that increased immune-system function correlates with less stress, anxiety, and depression. The same journal reported that among peripheral blood leukemia patients (and presumably among other cancer patients as well), psychological stress reduced levels of the cancer-fighting blood chemical interleukin-2. In related studies, relaxation and imagery were associated with decreased recurrence of ulcers; reduced anxiety, pain, and need for medication in femoral angiography procedures; and reduced hypertension.

Just as negative feelings and attitudes can lead to an impaired immune system that may increase one's suceptibility to cancer, so positive feelings and attitudes can be directed towards preventing cancer, or even causing cancer to regress. O. Carl Simonton, M.D., who, in the 1970s, pioneered the use of visual-imagery techniques for cancer patients, points out that cancer cells are not powerful, but are weak, deformed, and disorganized, having lost the ability to repair themselves or to perform any other complex function. This very weakness makes them vulnerable to many forms of treatment, including the body's own self-healing mechanisms.

In the laboratory, we have learned that white blood cells kill cancer. Through imagery, we can influence and direct our white blood cells to kill the cancer cells in our own bodies. It may be difficult or impossible to always feel positive, but it is always possible to *imagine* that we do. This technique can produce beneficial, healthy effects. Many of the same physiological benefits that one experiences through actual physical health can be achieved (and measured) by simply imagining healthy feelings.

Meditation and deep relaxation also enhance immune-system function. Meditation initiates a central nervous system response that is antithetical to the "fight-or-flight" response. Heart rate, blood pressure, blood flow, and breathing rates are lowered, as are levels of anxiety and stress as measured by increased skin resistance to electrical currents. In addition, meditation can specifically reduce cortisol levels.

A five-year study by Dr. David Orme-Johnson, which was published in *Psychosomatic Medicine* in 1989, showed a 50 percent overall reduction in health-care use among meditators. This overall reduction included decreases in the following areas:

- 87 percent in nervous system disorders
- 87 percent in heart disease
- 55 percent in tumors (malignant and benign)
- 30 percent in infectious diseases

Stress can also be reduced and immune-system function augmented by a high degree of social support. According to David Spiegel, M.D., of the Stanford University School of Medicine, being connected to people and having good personal relationships reduces death rates for all diseases. His own study at Stanford, reported in 1989, found that breast-cancer patients who joined a support group experienced an enhanced sense of purpose and self-worth, and they lived twice as long.

## WHAT YOU CAN DO ON A PERSONAL LEVEL

Become aware of the benefits of stress reduction on the immune system.

☐ Strengthen your immune system with such techniques as visual imagery, meditation, and deep relaxation (discussed in the first part of this chapter).

☐ Contact the following organizations for help in providing information on stress reduction:

Exceptional Cancer Patients
1302 Chapel Street
New Haven, CT 06511
(203) 865-8392

Simonton Cancer Center
Tapes and Literature Department
PO Box 1198
Azle, TX 76098
(800) 338-2360

☐ Read the following books on the subject of stress reduction.

*Awakening the Heart* edited by John Welwood. Boston: New Science Library, 1983.

*How to Meditate* by Lawrence LeShan. New York: Bantam Books, 1970.

*Minding the Body, Mending the Mind* by Joan Borysenko, Ph.D. New York: Bantam Books, 1988.

*Peace, Love and Healing* by Bernie Siegel. New York: Harper & Row, 1989.

*Peace of Mind: How You Can Learn to Meditate and Use the Power of Your Mind* by Dr. Ian Gawler. Garden City Park, NY: Avery Publishing Group, 1989.

*Quantum Healing* by Deepak Chopra, M.D. New York: Bantam Books, 1989.

*Seeking the Heart of Widsom: The Path of Insight Meditation* by Joseph Goldstein and Jack Kornfield. Boston, MA: Shambala Press, 1987.

# Chapter 35

# WORKPLACE HAZARDS

In 1775, the British surgeon Percival Pott observed a high incidence of cancer of the scrotum in chimney sweeps. He believed soot deposits that had lodged in the folds of the scrotum were the cause. This first report of cancer caused by conditions in the workplace led to further investigation of patterns of work-related disease, and ultimately, in the 1930s, to the identification of benzo-a-pyrene—a major component of chimney soot—as a powerful, coal-tar derived carcinogen.

Since Potts' observations, scientists have studied many groups of workers who suffer from specific work-related cancers. More human carcinogens have been identified by these studies than by any other means. For health and ethical reasons, suspected carcinogens are tested in clinical animal trials, not in human trials, and since there is not "sufficient evidence of human carcinogenisis, most cancer-causing substances are designated "animal carcinogens." However, the National Cancer Institute points out that substances causing cancer in one species usually cause cancer in others.

Cancer and other health problems in the workplace can result from chemicals used in commercial and industrial processes, from plant and equipment design, improper ventilation, atmospheric hazards, or "sick building syndrome"—buildings that have both poor ventilation and materials or furnishings that emit toxic fumes or gases. Some symptoms of "sick building syndrome" are dry or burning mucous membranes in the nose, eyes, and throat; sneezing; stuffy or runny nose; fatigue; lethargy; headache; dizziness; nausea; irritability; and personality change.

Exposure to benzidine, benzene, mustard gas, arsenic, vinyl chloride, asbestos, bis (chloromethyl) ether, chromium compounds, and coal-tar products has been linked to cancer in humans. Workers at high risk are those involved in the manufacturing of ethanol, isopropyl alcohol, paint, roofing materials, shoes, pharmaceuticals, textiles, and certain dyes.

Also at high risk to chemical exposure are workers in the steel, metal, rubber, and cable-making industries; iron-ore mining; creosoting; pipe coating; and nickel refining. Hairdressers, manicurists, dry cleaners, exterminators, medical students, medical-school instructors, laboratory-research technicians, farmers and farm workers, graphic artists, embalmers, gas-station attendants, construction workers, motor-vehicle inspectors, and operators of office machines are all at high cancer risk from chemical exposure.

Occupational Safety and Health Administration (OSHA) created the 1970 Occupational Safety and Health Act to "assure so far as possible every working man and woman in the nation safe and healthy working conditions." OSHA maintains and enforces health and safety standards that are established by the National Institute of Health and Safety (NIOSH); it keeps records of job-related injuries and illnesses and conducts research.

## WHAT YOU CAN DO ON A PERSONAL LEVEL

If you are employed in a high-risk workplace, be sure to know your rights. The following guidelines can help you lower occupational health risks.

☐ Ask your employer, or the manufacturer of chemicals to which you are exposed on the job, for the OSHA guidelines known as Material Safety Data Sheets (MSDSs) that are related to your specific workplace.

☐ Report hazards in the workplace by calling:

OSHA hotline
(800) 321-6742

☐ If you believe your job exposes you to hazardous chemicals, file a complaint with OSHA. If you belong to a union, ask a union official to sign the complaint. OSHA will schedule follow-up visits only if complaints are signed. Ask your union official to arrange for you to be there when the OSHA official arrives. To request an OSHA inspection while remaining anonymous, write to:

OSHA
Office of Information and Consumer Affairs
200 Constitution Avenue, NW – Room N3637
Washington, DC 20210

☐ To obtain records of OSHA's previous inspections of your company, tell them you are making a request under the Freedom of Information Act. Tell them you will pay searching and copying costs up to a certain amount of money, but that you want to be notified of costs beyond that amount. Send your request to OSHA (address above) by registered mail; by law they must respond within ten days.

☐ For information on health hazards of specific jobs and job sites, send a letter with your name, social security number, the name and location of the company for which you work, and your dates of employment to the following address. If you believe your workplace causes you and your coworkers to suffer from ill health, you can also request a NIOSH Health Hazard Evaluation.

NIOSH
4676 Columbia Parkway
Cincinnati, OH 45226
(800) 35-NIOSH
(513) 841-4382

☐ Ask your employer for your own exposure and medical records. Under OSHA's Access Standard, employers have to provide upon request all health records that have been kept during the past thirty years.

☐ Make a Freedom of Information request to the Environmental Protection Agency (EPA) to find out what chemicals and hazardous wastes are manufactured and generated at your workplace. Send your request to:

EPA
Freedom of Information Staff
401 M Street, SW – Room A 101
Washington, DC 20460

☐ To report or get records of your company's chemical releases (pollution emissions, spills, etc.), send a Freedom of Information Act request to:

National Response Center
2100 2nd Street, SW
Washington, DC 20593
(800) 424-8802
(202) 426-2675

☐ For a diagnostic evaluation of your workplace by a team of experienced engineers and microbiologists (the fee may range from $3,000 to $15,000), contact:

Healthy Buildings International, Inc.
  (HBI-USA)
10378 Democracy Lane
Fairfax, VA 22030
(703) 352-0102

☐ If you work in a small, non-union workplace, express any concerns to your coworkers and to your employer. Ask your employer to have an industrial hygienist assess and evaluate hazards. For a list of certified industrial-hygiene labs that can refer you to a qualified industrial hygienist, contact:

American Industrial Hygiene Association
PO Box 8390
345 White Pond Drive
Akron, OH 44320
(216) 873-2442

☐ If you work with printing processes, do not use petroleum-based inks that can expose you and your coworkers to heavy metals and volatile organic compounds. Use soy or vegetable-based inks. Some of the companies that sell these inks are listed below.

Alden & Ott Printing Ink Company
616 East Brook Drive
Arlington Heights, IL 60005
(708) 956-6830

Miller Cooper Ink Company
1601 Prospect Avenue
Kansas City, MO 64127
(816) 483-5020

Century Color
70 Colby Street
Medford, MA 02155
(617) 396-2970

Wikoff Color Corporation
PO Box W
Fort Mill, SC 29715
(803) 548-2210

☐ Additional information on hazards in the workplace is found in the following chapters: *Radiation in the Home, Nuclear Waste, Pesticides in the Home and Yard,* and *Smoking: Active and Passive.*

## HOW TO GET MORE INVOLVED

Your voice can make a difference. Following are some ways you can help bring about safer conditions in the workplace.

☐  Write to local, state, and federal legislators urging them to sponsor and support legislation to protect the health of workers in every occupation.

☐  Support the following organizations. They are committed to assuring a healthy atmosphere in the workplace. (Additional information on the organizations is found beginning on page 269.)

Public Citizen Health
  Research Group
2000 P Street, NW
Washington, DC 20036
(202) 872-0320

Safe Buildings Alliance
Metropolitan Square
Suite 1200
655 15th Street, NW
Washington, DC 20005
(202) 879-5120

Smoking Policy Institute
218 Broadway East
PO Box 20271
Seattle, WA 98102
(206) 324-4444

# YOU HAVE THE POWER

You have the power to take control of your own destiny in the battle against cancer. The risks are everywhere, but so are the tools that can reduce these risks.

There are four major ways you can bring about change. First, take responsibility for making the lifestyle changes that will lower your risks of getting cancer. Stack the odds in your favor.

Second, voice your concerns to the manufacturers of products that contain untested or cancer-causing substances. Express the same concerns to the store owners who sell the items. Your purchasing power can send a clear message. Explain that you will discontinue buying their products until they produce safer ones. In addition, express your concerns in writing to the appropriate federal agencies.

Administrator
Environmental Protection
  Agency
401 M Street, SW
Washington, DC  20460

Consumer Affairs
Food and Drug Adminis-
  tration
5600 Fishers Lane – HFE 88
Rockville, MD 20857

Third, write letters and make phone calls to your elected officials. Urge them to support bills and pass laws to improve and ensure public health and the health of the environment.

Elected officials know that for every phone call and letter received, there are thousands of other Americans who feel the same way. Addresses for the President and members of congress follow.

President
White House
1600 Pennsylvania Avenue, NW
Washington, DC 20500
(202) 456-1414

Congressperson
US House of Representatives
Washington, DC 20515
(202) 224-3121

Senator
US Senate
Washington, DC 20510
(202) 224-3121

Finally, join consumer groups and organizations that focus on public-interest issues. These independent, nonprofit organizations will keep you abreast of ongoing efforts and will give you a voice through their educational, legislative, and direct-action programs. Your financial support, time, and expertise can help play a critical role in the success of these organizations. Some groups are national, some regional, and others local. (Many national organizations can recommend local groups and affiliates.) On whatever level you choose to contribute, find a group whose goals are clearly stated. By joining a committed group, you can make a difference.

The following national organizations all champion public interests. Membership fees listed are for basic, individual one-year terms. Many organizations offer lower rates for students, senior citizens, and limited-income individuals. Some groups provide special group rates, as well.

Action on Smoking and
  Health (ASH)
2013 H Street, NW
Washington, DC 20006
(202) 659-4310

Founded in the late 1960s, this nonprofit, grassroots organization considers itself the "legal action arm" of the nonsmoking community. Lowering life-insurance rates for nonsmokers, and helping ban cigarette commercials on television are two examples of ASH's successful actions. ASH is supported entirely by contributions. For a donation of $15.00 or more, members receive a one-year subscription to *ASH Smoking and Health Review*, a bimonthly publication.

American Cancer Society
1599 Clifton Road, NE
Atlanta, GA 30329-4251
(800) ACS-2345
(404) 320-3333

The American Cancer Society is dedicated to conquering cancer through research, education, patient service, and rehabilitation. The Society is supported by gifts, grants, and individual contributions. There are no membership services.

American Lung Association
  (ALA)
1740 Broadway
New York, NY 10019
(212) 315-8700

The American Lung Association was founded in 1904 to fight tuberculosis. Today, under ALA's auspices, 129 separate state and local affiliates are dedicated to the prevention, cure, and control of all lung-related diseases and their causes. ALA offers public health-information materials, stop-smoking workshops, training and workshops for lung-disease sufferers, family asthma programs, and summer camps for children with asthma. ALA is also involved in political advocacy of lung health and clean air. Donations to the ALA are welcome. No membership services are provided.

American Oceans Campaign
  (AOC)
Suite 102
725 Arizona Avenue
Santa Monica, CA 90401
(310) 576-6162

Since its beginning in 1987, AOC has initiated projects and activities aimed at protecting our coasts and oceans. AOC activities have focused on protecting the coasts from offshore oil drilling while calling for a national energy policy, eliminating pollution of coastal waters, and preventing the loss of marine biodiversity through over-exploitation of living resources. Membership is $25.00. Members receive the quarterly AOC newsletter.

Americans for Nonsmokers'
 Rights (ANR)
2530 San Pablo Avenue, Suite J
Berkeley, CA 94702
(510) 841-3032

ANR is a nonprofit advocacy group created to develop legislative action that supports nonsmokers' rights to avoid involuntary exposure to secondhand smoke at work, in restaurants and public places, and on public transportation vehicles. ANR's educational arm, The American Nonsmokers' Rights Foundation (ANRF) develops educational programs for school children. Contributors receive *Update*, a quarterly newsletter.

Animal Protection Institute
 (API)
PO Box 22505
Sacramento, CA 95822
(916) 731-5521

API, founded in 1968, is dedicated to an "animal wonderful world." API offers extensive information on a wide range of animal topics including safety, health, and protection of the endangered. Information is available to anyone. Membership is $20.00. Members receive the quarterly magazine *Mainstream* and periodic newsletters.

Cancer Care, Inc.
1180 Avenue of the Americas
New York, NY 10036
(212) 221-3300

Cancer Care is a social service organization that offers counseling and guidance to help patients and families cope with the emotional and psychological consequences of cancer. Some financial assistance to eligible families is also provided. Cancer Care is a voluntary, independent, non-sectarian, nonprofit organization. It is supported by gifts, grants, and individual contributions. There are no membership services.

Center for Science in the
 Public Interest (CSPI)
Suite 300
1875 Connecticut Avenue, NW
Washington, DC 20009-5728
(202) 332-9110

CSPI, founded in 1971, focuses on four main areas: nutrition, food safety, organic agriculture, and alcohol policies. A donation of $19.95 entitles you to a one-year membership. Members are kept informed of current issues and activities through *The Nutrition Action Healthletter*, which is published ten times a year.

Citizens Clearinghouse for
 Hazardous Waste (CCHW)
PO Box 6086
Falls Church, VA 22040
(703) 237-CCHW

CCHW is a grassroots organization that helps communities organize effectively against hazardous and solid-waste problems. Focus is on clean air, soil, and drinking water. CCHW believes that people can and must speak for themselves in order for environmental justice to be best served. For a $25.00 yearly contribution, members receive the biannual newsletter *Everyone's Backyard.*

## Clean Water Action (CWA)
Suite 300
1320 18th Street, NW
Washington, DC 20036
(202) 457-1286

CWA is a national citizens organization committed to ensuring clean and safe water at an affordable cost, finding sensible solutions to the waste crisis, controlling the use and disposal of toxic chemicals, and protecting natural resources. CWA's educational arm, the Clean Water Action Fund, develops research and educational programs that complement lobbying activities and grassroots campaigns. For a yearly fee of $24.00, members receive the quarterly *Clean Water Action News* and periodic action-alert bulletins.

## Community Nutrition Institute (CNI)
2001 S Street, NW – Suite 500
Washington, DC 20009
(202) 462-4700

CNI, founded in 1970, is a public-interest group that monitors the federal government's nutrition and food-safety policies. CNI reports on government action through its weekly publication, *Nutrition Week.* There are no membership fees, but a one-year subscription to *Nutrition Week* costs $70.00.

## Consumers Union
Department NR (for contributions and subscription requests)
101 Truman Avenue
Yonkers, NY 10703-1057

Consumers Union, publisher of *Consumer Reports*, is a nonprofit organization established in 1936 to provide consumers with information and advice on goods, services, health and personal finance; and to initiate and cooperate with individual and group efforts to maintain and enhance the quality of life for consumers. Income is derived from the sale of *Consumer Reports* ($20.00 for yearly subscription), and from nonrestrictive, non-commercial contributions, grants, and fees.

## CURE Formaldehyde Poisoning Association
Attention: Connie Smrecek
9255 Lynnwood Road
Waconia, MN 55387
(612) 442-4665

Formed by formaldehyde-poisoning victims, CURE was established to keep the public informed about the hazards, treatment methods, and safe removal of formaldehyde. CURE is funded solely by private donations.

Earth Island Institute (EII)
300 Broadway – Suite 28
San Francisco, CA 94133-3312
(415) 788-3666

EII was founded in 1982 to develop innovative projects for the conservation, preservation, and restoration of the global environment.Membership is $25.00. Members receive the quarterly *Earth Island Journal* as well as periodic mailings about EII campaigns and events.

Environmental Action
  Foundation (EAF)
6930 Carroll Avenue
Takoma Park, MD 20912
(301) 891-1100

Through its support of grassroots action, EAF works to protect the Earth's resources for present and future generations. Goals of ongoing projects include strengthening environmental laws to protect drinking water, reduce toxic hazards, clean the air, and promote energy conservation. Yearly membership is $25.00; members receive the quarterly *Environmental Magazine*.

Environmental Defense Fund
  (EDF)
257 Park Avenue South
New York, NY 10010
(212) 505-2100

The EDF, founded in 1967, responds to emerging environmental concerns around the world. Ongoing EDF projects include the protection of natural resources; the defense of wildlife and wildlife habitats; the safeguarding of human health from toxic chemicals; and the development of comprehensive programs for waste reduction, re-use, recycling, and composting. Individual memberships are $15.00. Members receive the bimonthly *Environmental Defense Fund Newsletter*.

Food and Water, Inc.
Suite 613
225 Lafayette Street
New York, NY 10012
(800) EAT-SAFE
(212) 941-9340

Food and Water is a national organization working to prevent food irradiation. Yearly membership is $25.00. Members receive biannual newsletters, periodic updates, and action alerts on food irradiation.

Friends of the Earth (FOE)
218 D Street, SE
Washington, DC 20003
(202) 544-2600

Current projects of FOE include prevention of ozone-layer depletion; preservation of tropical forests; protection of oceans and coasts; monitoring global warming trends; finding solutions to problems of solid, hazardous, and nuclear waste; and promoting corporate responsibility.

Membership is $25.00. Members receive the monthly *Friends of the Earth Newsletter.*

## Gay Men's Health Crisis (GMHC)
129 West 20th Street
New York, NY 10011
(212) 807-6664
(212) 807-6655 (HOTLINE)

Founded in 1981, GMHC is the oldest and largest AIDS service organization. It provides direct service to the public through its information hotline. Legal and financial assistance, meal programs, and educational awareness programs are provided for men, women, and children with AIDS. GMHC accepts donations in any amount. There are no membership services.

## Grass Roots the Organic Way (GROW)
38 Llangollen Lane
Newton Square, PA 19073
(215) 353-2838

Founded by a pesticide-poisoning victim, GROW is a nonprofit organization formed to heighten public awareness of pesticide misuse; to influence legislation on local, state, and federal levels pertaining to the spraying of toxic pesticides in residential communities; and to create an information and resource network on safer alternatives to pesticide use. For a donation of $15.00, members receive current GROW literature and have access to the GROW information network.

## Greenpeace International
1436 U Street, NW
Washington, DC 20077
(202) 462-1177

Greenpeace is a nonprofit, grassroots organization that fights pollution of the Earth's air, water, land, and wildlife. Goals include the ending of industrial pollution, the protection of whales being killed for scientific research, and a ban on driftnet fishing, which kills dolphins, seals, and marine birds. Membership is $20.00. Members receive the quarterly newsletter *Greenpeace* and other action-alert releases.

## Group Against Smoking Pollution (GASP)
25 Deaconess Road
Boston, MA 02215
(617) 266-2088

GASP publicizes the harmful effects of tobacco on nonsmokers; promotes laws and court decisions that protect rights of nonsmokers; helps establish smoke-free workplaces; and encourages the enforcement of no-smoking laws. Yearly membership is $20.00. Members receive quarterly issues of The GASP Newsletter.

## Household Hazardous Waste Project (HHWP)
1031 E. Battlefield – Suite 214
Springfield, MO 65807
(417) 889-5000

HHWP is a nonprofit project of the University of Missouri Extension System. HHWP provides training, consultation, educational materials, and a referral and information service for concerns about household hazardous products. There is no membership service.

INFORM, Inc.
381 Park Avenue South
New York, NY 10016
(212) 689-4040

Founded in 1974, INFORM is a research organization whose main focus is on urban air quality and the prevention/reduction of solid and hazardous waste. Through its books and reports, INFORM provides background research for legislators, business people, and consumer groups. For a yearly donation of $25.00 or more, members receive the quarterly newsletter *INFORM Reports* and discounts on other INFORM publications.

Mothers Against Drunk
  Driving (MADD)
PO Box 541688
Dallas, TX 75354-1688
(214) 744-MADD

Mothers Against Drunk Driving, founded in 1980, is a nonprofit, grassroots organization with more than 400 chapters nationwide. MADD firmly believes that drunk driving is a violent crime. The group's mission is to stop drunk driving and to support the victims of this crime. Membership is $20.00 (no dues for victims). Members receive *MADD in Action*, the group's national newsletter, two to three times each year.

National Alliance of Breast
  Cancer Organizations
  (NABCO)
Second Floor
1180 Avenue of the Americas
New York, NY 10036

NABCO provides individuals and health organizations with accurate, current information on all aspects of breast cancer. NABCO is also active in efforts to influence public and private health policy on issues that directly pertain to breast cancer. Membership is $40.00. Members receive quarterly issues of *NABCO News*, NABCO's *Resource List* of informative materials, and special mailings.

National Center for Environmental Health Strategies
  (NCEHS)
1100 Rural Avenue
Voorhees, NJ 08043
(609) 429-5358

The NCEHS provides clearinghouse, technical, referral, support, and advocacy services for the public, especially for those with environmentally and occupationally induced illnesses. The goals of NCEHS include the elimination or minimization of toxic exposures in the home, workplace, school, and outdoor environment. Membership is $15.00. Members receive the quarterly NCEHS newsletter entitled *The Delicate Balance*, discounts on the Center's publications, and use of its services.

## National Coalition Against the Misuse of Pesticides (NCAMP)
701 E Street, SE – Suite 200
Washington, DC 20003
(202) 543-5450

NCAMP, founded in 1981, promotes least-toxic methods of pest control in and around the home, in public facilities, and in agriculture. NCAMP advocates policies that protect the public from pesticide exposure, and it assists community organizations with alternative methods of pest control. Yearly membership fee is $25.00. Members receive five issues of *Pesticides and You.*

## National Council on Alcoholism and Drug Dependence (NCADD)
12 West 21st Street
New York, NY 10010
(212) 206-6770
NCADD, founded in 1944, works to prevent alcohol and drug abuse, and to assist those who are already suffering from these addictions. Through affiliate-sponsored community-based prevention and education programs, national public-awareness campaigns, and public

policy and prevention initiatives, NCADD has helped change the ways our society views and addresses problems associated with drug and alcohol addiction. Membership is $100.00. Members receive the quarterly *Update* and periodic releases.

## National Women's Health Network
1325 G Street, NW
Washington, DC 20005
(202) 347-1140

National Women's Health Network advocates better federal health policies for women. Considered an FDA watchdog (especially on hormone-related issues), this group is also a clearinghouse for women's health information. For a $25.00 yearly donation, members receive six issues of *The Network News*, a newsletter with pertinent updates and information on women and health.

## Natural Resources Defense Council (NRDC)
40 West 20th Street
New York, NY 10011
(212) 727-2700

Founded in 1970, the NRDC works to protect our water, air, and food supplies through effective legislation, advocacy, and research. NRDC promotes conservation, environmentally safe energy sources, and energy-efficient standards. This organization has also spearheaded programs that address issues of global warming, the proliferation of nuclear weapons, and the protection of the ozone layer. For a $10.00 contribution, members receive two quarterly publications, *The Amicus Journal* and *Newsline*. Members also receive alerts and updates on high-priority projects.

Northwest Coalition for Alternatives to Pesticides (NCAP)
PO Box 1393
Eugene, OR 97440
(503) 344-5044

NCAP provides assistance in developing model policies to protect the groundwater, the food supply, and the forest watersheds from pesticide contamination. In addition, NCAP establishes pesticide management programs, educates communities on safe alternatives to pesticides, refers pesticide-exposure victims to agencies that provide appropriate recourse, and organizes community pesticide-policy reform projects. Yearly membership is $25.00. Members receive the quarterly *Journal of Pesticide Reform* and updates on reform projects and policy initiatives from across the country.

Nuclear Information &
Resource Service (NIRS)
1424 16th Street, NW – 601
Washington, DC 20036
(202) 328-0002

NIRS was founded in 1978. Through educating the public and by its lobbying activities, NIRS promotes safe energy alternatives to fossil fuel and nuclear power plants. NIRS allies itself with the growing grassroots movement against all unnecessary toxic substances in the environment. For a donation in any amount, contributors receive periodic regulatory alerts. For a $35.00 donation, members receive *The Nuclear Monitor*, a biweekly newsletter.

People for the Ethical Treatment of Animals (PETA)
PO Box 42516
Washington, DC 20015-0516
(301) 770-7444

Founded in 1980, PETA is dedicated to establishing and defending the rights of all animals, and operates under the simple principle that animals are not ours to eat, wear, experiment on, or use for entertainment. PETA works through public education, research and investigations, legislation, direct action, and grassroots organizing. Membership is $15.00. Members receive the quarterly *PETA News* and periodic action alerts and updates.

Physicians for Social
Responsibility (PSR)
Suite 810
1000 16th Street, NW
Washington, DC 20036
(202) 785-3777

PSR, founded in 1961, is a national, consumer-oriented organization committed to arms control and to help safeguard the public health from radioactive and toxic pollutants. PSR welcomes contributions but provides no membership services.

Project Inform (PI)
Room 220
1965 Market Street
San Francisco, CA 94103
(800) 822-7422
(800) 334-7422 (in California)

Established in 1985, PI provides AIDS treatment service information through its hotline. This organization advocates early intervention and treatment of HIV carriers. Project Inform publishes *PI Perspectives*, a free newsletter dealing with the latest HIV/AIDS treatment information. Funded through private donations, PI welcomes contributions in any amount.

Public Citizen
2000 P Street, NW
Washington, DC 20036
(202) 833-3000

Founded in 1971 by Ralph Nader, Public Citizen fights for consumer rights in the marketplace, safe products, a healthy environment in the workplace, clean and safe energy sources, and government and corporate accountability. Funding comes from the sale of its publications and from individual donations. For a contribution of $20.00 or more, members receive a one-year subscription to *Public Citizen*, a bimonthly publication.

Radioactive Waste Campaign
7 West Street
Warwick, NY 10990
(914) 986-1115
(718) 387-8786

Radioactive Waste Campaign promotes greater public awareness of the dangers to human health and the environment from the production, transportation, and storage of radioactive waste. This organization provides a wide range of information through its books, fact sheets, slide shows, videos, and its quarterly newspaper called *The Waste Paper*. Membership is $20.00. Members receive a discount on publications and a subscription to *The Waste Paper*.

Renew America
Suite 710
1400 Sixteenth Street, NW
Washington, DC 20036
(202) 232-2252

Renew America is a national clearinghouse for proposed environmental solutions. Renew America's *Searching for Success* identifies and verifies successful programs created by individuals and organizations throughout the United States for environmental protection, enhancement, and restoration. Certificates of environmental achievement are awarded to designated programs, which are described in the *Environmental Success Index* directory. Membership is $25.00. Members receive the quarterly newsletter *Renew America Reports*, as well as discounts on the group's other publications.

Safe Buildings Alliance
Suite 1200
Metropolitan Square
655 Fifteenth Street, NW
Washington, DC 20005
(202) 879-5120

Founded in 1984 to promote a reasoned, scientifically sound approach to the issue of asbestos in buildings, Safe Buildings Alliance advocates sound asbestos-inspection techniques, and practical alternatives to dangerous asbestos removal. This group also advocates the establishment of training, certification, and work-practice requirements for asbestos workers. Safe Buildings Alliance provides scientific studies and fact sheets, and also advises people on communicating their concerns to elected public officials.

SANE/FREEZE
1819 H Street, NW – Suite 640
Washington, DC 20006-3603
(202) 862-9740

The primary goals of SANE/FREEZE are nuclear disarmament, banning the production of radioactive fissile materials, and ending global arms trade. SANE/FREEZE operates on the national level and also organizes grassroots activists.

Membership is $25.00. Members receive the quarterly *SANE/FREEZE NEWS* and periodic updates on their current projects.

Sierra Club
730 Polk Street
San Francisco, CA 94109
(415) 923-5653

Founded in 1892, the Sierra Club promotes the conservation of the natural environment by influencing public-policy decisions. This group campaigns on the national, state, and local levels for the responsible use of the Earth's ecosystems and resources. Yearly membership is $35.00. Members receive the magazine *Sierra*, which is published six times a year.

Smoking Policy Institute (SPI)
914 East Jefferson
PO Box 20271
Seattle, WA 98102
(216) 324-4444

SPI is a nonprofit corporation that helps organizations in creating healthy, smoke-free environments for employees. Through information packages, products, and consulting services, the Institute helps develop and implement customized smoking-control policies.

U.S. Public Interest Research Group (U.S.PIRG)
215 Pennsylvania Avenue, SE
Washington, DC 20003
(202) 546-9707

U.S.PIRG is the national lobbying office for state PIRGs around the country. It conducts independent research and lobbies for national environmental and consumer protections. This group also campaigns against toxic chemicals, lobbies for energy efficiency, supports recycling and waste-reduction programs, and alerts consumers against unsafe products. U.S.PIRG is funded by donations from individual citizens. For a contribution of $15.00 or more, members receive the newsletter *U.S.PIRG Citizen Agenda*.

Union of Concerned Scientists (UCS)
26 Church Street
Cambridge, MA 02236
(617) 547-5552

UCS was founded in 1969 to bring focus to environmental issues such as damage from fossil fuels, energy efficiency, and renewable energy sources. USC conducts research and works with local, state, and federal governments and business communities to bring about sensible change.

Membership is $20.00. Members receive the quarterly *Nucleus Journal* and periodic bulletins on UCS activities.

Y-ME
National Organization for Breast Cancer Information and Support
18220 Harwood Avenue
Homewood, IL 60430
(708) 799-8338

Y-ME is a national information and support group for people concerned with breast-cancer issues. Y-ME staffs a national hotline and provides many complimentary services including pretreatment counseling; early-detection workshops; a wig and prosthesis bank; and referrals on mammogram facilities, treatment and research hospitals, breast specialists, and nationwide support programs. Membership is $15.00. Members receive the bimonthly *Y-ME Hotline* and periodic mailings. *(Services are not limited to members; they are available to anyone.)*

# REFERENCES

## Introduction

Brody, Jane E. "Natural Chemicals Now Called Major Cause of Disease." *The New York Times*, April 26, 1988.

*Everything Doesn't Cause Cancer.* Bethesda, MD: United States Department of Health, Education and Welfare, Public Health Service. National Institutes of Health, March 1990.

*Good News, Better News, Best News . . . Cancer Prevention.* Bethesda, MD: United States Department of Health. National Cancer Institute, Publication 84-2671.

"Preventing Cancer." *Nutrition Action Health Letter*, Vol. 14, No. 6, July–August, 1987.

Warren, Jacqueline M. "Cancer Risk Assessment." Washington, DC: *NRDC Newsline*, April 1991.

## Chapter 1 /    Additives in Food

Burros, Marion. "U.S. Food Regulation: Tales from a Twilight Zone." *The New York Times*, June 10, 1987.

Dadd, Debra Lynn. *Nontoxic, Natural and Earthwise.* Los Angeles, CA: Jeremy P. Tarcher, 1990.

*Eating Clean: Overcoming Food Hazards.* Washington, DC: Center for the Study of Responsive Law, 1988.

"EPA Sets Legal Strategy to Cut Delaney Clause." *Nutrition Weekly*, May 10, 1990.

Jacobson, Michael F., PhD. *The Complete Eater's Digest and Nutrition Scoreboard.* Garden City, NY: Anchor Press/Doubleday, 1985.

———*Safe Food: Eating Wisely in a Risky World.* Venice, CA: Living Planet Press, 1991.

———"Undoing Delaney: FDA Allows Free Use of Dangerous Additives." *Nutrition Action Healthletter*, September–October 1985.

Lehmann, Phyllis. "More Than You Ever Thought You Would Know About Food Additives." *FDA Consumer*, February 1982.
*The Complete Book of Cancer Prevention.* Emmaus, PA: Rodale Press, 1988.
Winter, Ruth. *Cancer-Causing Agents.* New York: Crown Publishers, 1979.

## Chapter 2 / *Aflatoxin*

"Aflatoxin and Cancer." *Nutrition Week*, April 26, 1991.
"Aflatoxin-contaminated Corn Found in Midwest; Health Danger Possible." *Nutrition Week*, September 9, 1988.
"Aflatoxin in Corn Supply Threatens Grain Exports and Domestic Food Stocks." *Nutrition Week*, August 24, 1989.
Burros, Marion. "U.S. Food Regulation: Tales from a Twilight Zone." *The New York Times*, June 6, 1987.
"FDA Asked to Develop New Aflatoxin Rules." *Nutrition Week*, July 27, 1989.
Jacobson, Michael F., PhD. *The Complete Eater's Digest and Nutrition Scoreboard.* Garden City, NY: Anchor Press/Doubleday, 1985.
Jensen, Dr. Bernard and Mark Anderson. *Empty Harvest.* Garden City Park, NY: Avery Publishing Group, 1990.
McKelway, Ben, ed. *Guess What's Coming to Dinner.* Washington, DC: Center for Science in the Public Interest, March 1987.
"New Aflatoxin Outbreak Hits 3 Southern States." September 20, 1990.
"The Drought's Toxic Harvest." *Time*, October 31, 1988.
Winter, Ruth. *Cancer-Causing Agents.* New York: Crown Publishers, 1979.

## Chapter 3 / *Alcohol*

"Alcohol and Cancer." *Lancet*, March 17, 1990.
Burros, Marion. "U.S. Food Regulation: Tales from a Twilight Zone." *The New York Times*, June 6, 1987.
"Chemical is Said to Taint Alcohol." *The New York Times*, December 14, 1987.
Dadd, Debra Lynn. *Nontoxic and Natural.* Los Angeles, CA: Jeremy P. Tarcher, 1984.
*Eating Clean: Overcoming Food Hazards.* Washington, DC: Center for the Study of Responsive Law, 1988.
Farrow, D.C. et al. "Risk of pancreatic cancer in relation to medical history and the use of tobacco, alcohol and coffee." *International Journal of Cancer*, May 1990.
Fisher, Lawrence M. "Lead Levels in Many Wines Exceed U.S. Standards for Water." *The New York Times*, August 2, 1991.
——"Organic Wines Enter the Mainstream." *The New York Times*, November 19, 1991.
Gold, Mark S., MD. *The Facts About Drugs and Alcohol.* New York: Bantam Books, 1986.
Leary, Warren E. "Wine Makers Agree to Reduce Urethane." *The New York Times*, January 25, 1988.

Mitchell, Charles P. and Michael F. Jacobson, PhD. *Tainted Booze.* Washington, DC: Center for Science in the Public Interest, December 1987.
Nomura, A. et. al. "Smoking, alcohol and hair dye use in cancer of the lower urinary tract." *American Journal of Epidemiology,* June 1990.
Prial, Frank J. "Wine talk." *The New York Times,* February 20, 1991.
Yoder, Barbara. *The Recovery Resource Book.* New York: Simon & Schuster, 1990.

## Chapter 4 / *Caffeine*

Brody, Jane E. "Rise in Soft Drink Consumption." *The New York Times,* May 13, 1987.
————"Scientists Seeking Possible Wonder Drugs in Tea." *The New York Times,* March 14, 1991.
*Eating Clean: Overcoming Food Hazards.* Washington, DC: Center for the Study of Responsive Law, 1988.
Farrow, D.C. et al. "Risk of pancreatic cancer in relation to medical history and the use of tobacco, alcohol and coffee." *International Journal of Cancer,* May 1990.
Hearne, Shelley A. "Harvest of Unknowns: Pesticide Contamination in Imported Foods." Washington, DC: Natural Resources Defense Council, 1984.
"Lawsuit Seeks to Prohibit Use of Carcinogen Methylene Chloride in Decaffeinated Coffee." *Health Research Group Health Letter,* July–August 1988.
Weisskopf, Michael. "FDA Admits Laxity in Testing Food Imports." *The Washington Post,* May 1, 1987.

## Chapter 5 / *Dietary Fat*

Blume, Elaine. "Why Oxidized Fats are in Your Food and Why You Wish They Weren't." *Nutrition Action Health Letter,* December 1987.
Brody, Jane E. "Huge Study of Diet Indicts Fat and Meat." *The New York Times,* May 8, 1990.
Burros, Marion. "A Change in Cooking Oil Can Improve Your Diet." *The New York Times,* December 9, 1987.
Carroll, Kenneth K. "Dietary Fats and Cancer." *American Journal of Clinical Nutrition,* April 1991.
Deschner, Eleanor E., PhD. "The effect of dietary omega-3 fatty acids (fish oil) on azoxymethenol-induced focal areas of dysplasia and colon tumor incidence." *Cancer: A Journal of the American Cancer Society,* December 1, 1990.
"Fish Oil: Fad or Find?" *Nutrition Action Health Letter,* March 1989.
Gittleman, Ann Louise. *Beyond Pritikin.* New York: Bantam Books, 1988.
Harrison, Lewis. *Making Fats and Oils Work For You.* Garden City Park, NY: Avery Publishing Group, 1990.
Holm, L.E. et al. "Dietary habits and prognostic factors in breast cancer." *Journal of the National Cancer Institute,* August 16, 1989.

Howe, G.R. et al. "A cohort study of fat intake and risk of breast cancer." *Journal of the National Cancer Institute*, March 6, 1991.

Liebman, Bonnie. "Clues to Colon Cancer." *Nutrition Action Health Letter*, March 1990.

————"What, Meat Worry?" *Nutrition Action Newsletter*, June 1991.

O'Connor, T.P. et al. "Effects of dietary omega-3 and omega-6 fatty acids on development of azaserine-induced preneoplastic lesions in rat pancreas." *Journal of the National Cancer Institute*, June 7, 1989.

"Official Blows Whistle on Pyramid Cancellation." *Nutrition Week*, November 22, 1991.

Passwater, Richard A., PhD. *Evening Primrose Oil*. New Canaan, CT: Keats Publishing, 1981.

Pjuric, Z. et al. "Effects of a low fat diet on levels of oxidation damage to DNA in peripheral nucleatal blood cells." *Journal of the National Cancer Institute*, June 5, 1991.

Schatzkin, Arthur, Peter Greenwald, David Byar, and Carolyn K. Clifford. "The Dietary Fat-Breast Cancer Hypothesis is Alive." *Journal of the American Medical Association*, June 9, 1989.

Schilder, Jackie. "Holistic Currents." *Holistic Living*, July–August 1990.

"Seafood fatty acids may lower cancer risk." *Journal of the National Cancer Institute*, October 18, 1989.

Simone, Charles B., MD. *Cancer and Nutrition*. Garden City Park, NY: Avery Publishing Group, 1992.

Snider, Mike. "More evidence that diet can cut cancer risk." *USA Today*, April 23, 1991.

*The Complete Book of Cancer Prevention*. Emmaus, PA: Rodale Press, 1988.

"USDA's Pyramid Scheme." *Nutrition Action Newsletter*, June 1991.

**Chapter 6 /  *Dietary Imbalance***

Brewster, Letitia and Michael Jacobson, PhD. *The Changing American Diet: a Chronicle of American Eating Habits from 1910 to 1980*. Washington, DC: Center for Science in the Public Interest, 1983.

*Diet, Nutrition and Cancer Prevention: A Guide to Food Choices*. National Institutes of Health, 1987.

*Diet, Nutrition and Cancer Prevention: The Good News*. National Cancer Institute Publication 87-2878, 1987.

"Intriguing Studies Link Nutrition to Immunity." *The New York Times*, March 21, 1989.

Jacobson, Michael F., PhD. *The Complete Eater's Digest and Nutrition Scoreboard*. Garden City, NY: Anchor Press/Doubleday, 1985.

————*Safe Food: Eating Wisely in a Risky World*. Venice, CA: Living Planet Press, 1991.

"Official Blows Whistle on Pyramid Cancellation." *Nutrition Week*, November 22, 1991.

*Population Strategies for Blood Cholesterol Reduction*. National Institutes of Health Publication No. 90–3046, November 1990.

Simone, Charles B., MD. *Cancer and Nutrition.* Garden City Park, NY: Avery Publishing Group, 1992.

**Chapter 7 /    *Irradiation of Food***

Dadd, Debra Lynn. *Nontoxic, Natural and Earthwise.* Los Angeles, CA: Jeremy P. Tarcher, 1990.

Fazzino, Jean. "Food Irradiation." *Radioactive Waste Campaign (RWC) Waste Paper,* Summer 1988.

"Food Irradiation: A technique for Preserving and Improving the Safety of Food." World Health Organization, Geneva, 1988.

"Food Irradiation Update." *CANAH Health Rights Advocate,* Summer 1988.

Herbst, Walter. "Irradiation of Foods: Health Risks Extrapolated from Incalculable Health Risks by Food Irradiation." *Coalition for Alternatives in Nutrition and Health Care,* 1988.

*Irradiated Foods.* New York: The American Council on Science and Health, 1988 (rev.).

"Irradiation in the Production, Processing and Handling of Food: Final Rule." Federal Register, 21 CFR Part 179, April 18, 1986.

"Irrational Irradiation." *Science for the People,* July–August 1988.

"Is Irradiation Safe or Necessary?" *Health Research Group Health Letter,* March–April 1985.

"New Hope or False Promise: Biotechnology and Third World Agriculture." *International Coalition for Development Action,* Brussels, Belgium, 1987.

Radelat, A. "Wired: Are Power Lines and Household Appliances Hazardous to Your Health?" *Public Citizen,* May–June 1991.

"Report on the Safety and Wholesomeness of Irradiated Foods." Advisory Committee on Irradiated and Novel Foods, United Kingdom, March 1986.

Schechter, Steven R. with T. Monte. *Fighting Irradiation with Foods, Herbs, and Vitamins.* Brookline, MA: East West Health Books, 1988.

"The Attacks on the Delaney Amendment." *Food Irradiation Alert,* Vol. 2, No. 3, December 1987.

Webb, Tony, Tim Lang, and Kathleen Tucker. *Food Irradiation: Who Wants It?* Northamptonshire, England: Thorsons Publishing Group, 1987.

"What Has Been Done to Fight Food Irradiation?" *Health Research Group Health Letter,* November–December 1986.

Willis, Camille. " Gamma Gourmet: Food Irradiation Sparks Controversy." *The NYPIRG Activist,* Fall 1987.

**Chapter 8 /    *Lack of Dietary Fiber***

Balch, James F., MD and Phyllis A. Balch, CNC. *Prescription for Nutritional Healing.* Garden City Park, NY: Avery Publishing Group, 1990.

Brody, Jane E. "Huge Study of Diet Indicts Fat and Meat." *The New York Times,* May 8, 1990.

*Diet, Nutrition and Cancer Prevention: A Guide to Food Choices.* United States Department of Health and Human Services, National Cancer Institute Publication 87-2878, May 1987.

"Evidence of Protective Effects of Wheat Fiber Grows." *Journal of the National Cancer Institute,* November 20, 1991.

Friend, Tim. "Fiber may lower breast cancer risk." *USA Today,* April 3, 1991.

Gittleman, Ann Louise. *Beyond Pritikin.* New York: Bantam Books, 1988.

Holm, L.E. et al. "Dietary habits and prognostic factors in breast cancer." *Journal of the National Cancer Institute,* August 16, 1989.

Jacobson, Michael F., PhD. *The Complete Eater's Digest and Nutrition Scoreboard.* Garden City, NY: Anchor Press/Doubleday, 1985.

Kushi, Michio. *Cancer Prevention Diet.* New York: St. Martin's Press, 1983.

Liebman, Bonnie. "Clues to Colon Cancer." *Nutrition Action Health Letter,* March 1990.

Simone, Charles B., MD. *Cancer and Nutrition.* Garden City Park, NY: Avery Publishing Group, 1992.

"The Facts About Fruit." *Nutrition Action Health Letter,* Vol. 14, No. 6, July–August 1987.

Trock, B. et al. "Dietary Fiber, vegetables, and colon cancer: a critical review and meta-analysis of the epidemiologic evidence." *Journal of the National Cancer Institute,* April 18, 1990.

Winter, Ruth. *Cancer-Causing Agents.* New York: Crown Publishers, 1979.

**Chapter 9 /    Lack of Vitamins and Minerals**

Adams, R. and F. Murray. *Improving Your Health with Vitamin C.* New York: Larchmont Books, 1978.

Balch, James F., MD, and P. Balch, CNC. *Prescription for Nutritional Healing.* Garden City Park, NY: Avery Publishing Group, 1990.

Barone, Jeanine. "Can Diet Protect Your Immune System?" *Nutrition Action Health Letter,* August 1988.

Bland, Jeffrey S., PhD. "RDA Update." *East West,* July 1990.

Block, Gladys. "Vitamin C and cancer prevention: the epidemiologic evidence." *American Journal of Clinical Nutrition,* January 1991.

Bresnick, Jan. "Foods That Heal." *Prevention,* December 1987.

Brody, Jane E. "Intriguing Studies Link Nutrition to Immunity." *The New York Times,* March 21, 1989.

————"Personal Health: New Research Bolsters Long-Held Belief that Vitamin E Can Provide an Array of Reliefs." *The New York Times,* April 27, 1989.

————"The Effort to Prevent Cancer Moves to New Stage." *The New York Times,* January 9, 1989.

Cameron, E. and L. Pauling. *Cancer and Vitamin C.* Menlo Park, CA: Linus Pauling Institute for Science and Medicine, 1979.

Colbin, Annemarie. *Food and Healing.* New York: Ballantine Books, 1986.

Garland, Dr. Cedric and Dr. Frank Garland. "The Calcium/Cancer Connection." *Prevention,* January 1988.

Howe, G.R. et al. "Dietary factors and risk of breast cancer: combined analysis of 12 case-controlled studies." *Journal of the National Cancer Institute,* April 4, 1990.

Kelly, Dennis. "Vitamin C fosters healthier sperm." *USA Today,* December 16, 1991.

Klein, Morton and C. Perlmutter. "Vitamin C Against Cancer." *Prevention,* March 1991.

Knekt, Paul et al. "Vitamin E and cancer prevention." *American Journal of Clinical Nutrition,* January 1991.

LeMarchand, L. et al. "Vegetable consumption and lung cancer: a population-based case control study in Hawaii." *Journal of the National Cancer Institute,* August 2, 1989.

Lieberman, Shari and Nancy Bruning. *The Real Vitamin and Mineral Book.* Garden City Park, NY: Avery Publishing Group, 1990.

Malesky, Gale. "Food Factors that Stop Cancer: Best News, Best Bets." *Prevention,* October 1987.

Malone, Winifred F. "Studies evaluating antioxidants and beta-carotene as chemopreventives." *American Journal of Clinical Nutrition,* January 1991.

Mayer, J.A. *Diet for Living.* New York: Pocket Books, 1977.

Mindell, Earl. *Vitamin Bible.* New York: Warner Books, 1985.

"No Zinc Without Copper." *Nutrition Action Newsletter,* June 1991.

Pais, Ray C., MD, et al. "Abnormal vitamin $B_6$ status in childhood leukemia." *Cancer—A Journal of the American Cancer Society,* December 1, 1990.

Passwater, R.A. *Cancer and its Nutritional Therapies.* New Canaan, CT: Pivot Original Health Books, 1978.

Simone, Charles B., MD. *Cancer and Nutrition.* Garden City Park, NY: Avery Publishing Group, 1992.

Stahelin, H.B. et al. "Beta-carotene and cancer prevention: the Basel study." *American Journal of Clinical Nutrition.* January 1991.

Tannenbaum, Steven R. et al. "Inhibition of nitrosamine formation by ascorbic acid." *American Journal of Clinical Nutrition,* January 1991.

*The Complete Book of Cancer Prevention.* Emmaus, PA: Rodale Press, 1988.

"Vitamin C: How it may protect against cancer." *Journal of the National Cancer Institute,* March 20, 1991.

Weisburger, John H. "Nutritional approach to cancer prevention with emphasis on vitamins, antioxidants and carotenoids." *American Journal of Clinical Nutrition,* January 1991.

"Why We Need Nutritional Supplements." *Health Rights Advocate,* March 1990.

**Chapter 10 /** *Meat, Poultry, and Fish*

Brody, Jane E. "Huge Study of Diet Indicts Fat and Meat." *The New York Times,* May 8, 1990.

Burros, Marion. "Eating Well: Beach Pollution This Summer is Apparently Scaring a Lot of People Away from Seafood." *The New York Times,* August 10, 1988.

————"Fat's in the Fire: A Guide for the Wary." *The New York Times,* March 27, 1991.

————"Grilling, Frying and Broiling Are Found to be Links in the Meat-Cancer Connection." *The New York Times,* March 27, 1991.

————"Study of Retail Fish Markets Finds Wide Contamination and Mislabeling." *The New York Times,* January 16, 1992.

————"U.S. Food Regulation: Tales from a Twilight Zone." *The New York Times,*July 10, 1987.

*Eating Clean: Overcoming Food Hazards.* Washington, DC: Center for the Study of Responsive Law, 1988.

"Fish Advisory." Wisconsin Department of Natural Resources, Division of Health, April 1991.

"Fishing and Pollution Imperil Coastal Fish, Several Studies Find." *The New York Times,* July 16, 1991.

*Hidden Hazards of Meat and Poultry: A Consumer's Guide.* Washington, DC: Natural Resources Defense Council, 1988.

"Is Our Fish Fit to Eat?" *Consumer Reports,* February, 1992.

Jacobson, Michael F., PhD. *The Complete Eater's Guide and Nutrition Scoreboard.* Garden City, NY: Anchor Press/Doubleday, 1985.

Kantor, Michael. "Dangerous Dregs in the Deep." *Sierra,* May–June 1988.

Luoma, Jon R. "Study Questions Adequacy of Warnings About Tainted Fish." *The New York Times,* February 28, 1989.

Lefferts, Lisa Y. "Good Fish . . . Bad Fish." *Nutrition Action Health Letter,* Vol. 15, No. 8, October 1988.

McKelway, Ben, ed. *Guess What's Coming to Dinner?* Washington, DC: Center for Science in the Public Interest, March 1987.

"Scientists Question Safety of Fish Consumption." *Journal of the National Cancer Institute,* November 1, 1989.

Snider, Mike. "More evidence that diet can cut cancer risk." *USA Today,* April 23, 1991.

## Chapter 11 /    *Pesticides in Foods*

*A Citizen's Guide to Pesticides.* United States Environmental Protection Agency, September 1987.

*Action on Pesticides.* San Francisco, CA: Sierra Club, May 1984.

"Animals, Toxics and Us." *Garbage: The Practical Journal for the Environment,* July–August 1991.

Burros, Marion. "New Urgency Fuels Effort to Improve Safety of Food." *The New York Times,* May 7, 1990.

————"That Blemished Product May Be the Most Healthful to Eat." *The New York Times,* April 3, 1991.

Carlson, Margaret. "Do You Dare to Eat a Peach?" *Time,* March 27, 1989.

Dover, Michael. "Getting Off the Pesticide Treadmill." *Technology Review,* November–December 1985.

*Eating Clean: Overcoming Food Hazards.* Washington, DC: Center for the Study of Responsive Law, 1988.

Garland, Anne Witte. *For Our Kids' Sake: How to Protect Your Child Against Pesticides in Food.* Washington, DC: Natural Resources Defense Council, 1989.

"Good News." *Cancer Forum*, Winter 1991.

Harris, Stephanie G. *Grow It Safely: Pesticide Control Without Poisons.* Washington, DC: Public Citizen Health Research Group, 1975.

Lefferts, Lisa Y. "Pass the Pesticides." *Nutrition Action Health Letter*, Vol. 16, No. 3, April 1989.

Milius, Susan. "Pesticide SOS." *Organic Gardening*, October 1987.

Montgomery, Anne. "America's Pesticide-Permeated Food." *Nutrition Action Health Letter*, Vol. 14, No. 5, June 1987.

Mott, Lawrie. *Pesticides in Food: What the Public Needs to Know.* Washington, DC: Natural Resources Defense Council, March 15, 1984.

Mott, Lawrie and Karen Snyder. *Pesticide Alert: A Guide to Pesticides in Fruits and Vegetables.* San Francisco, CA: Sierra Club Books, 1987.

*Pesticide Safety: Myths and Facts.* Washington, DC: National Campaign Against the Misuse of Pesticides, 1988.

Reynolds, Barbara. " 'Cide means kill; that's exactly what pesticides do." *USA Today*, April 22, 1991.

Roueche, Berton. "Annals of Medicine: The Fumigation Chamber." *The New Yorker*, January 4, 1988.

Stiak, Jim. "Pesticides and Secret Agents." *Sierra*, May–June 1988.

Vogel, Shawna. "Biowaste: Quiet Hazard." *Not Man Apart*, September–October 1989.

"Waxing Scientific on Fruit." *New York Life*, November 22, 1987.

Weisskopf, Michael. "FDA Admits Laxity in Testing Food Imports." *The Washington Post*, May 1, 1987.

Zwerdling, Michael. "The Pesticide Treadmill." *The Environmental Journal*, September 1987.

## Chapter 12 / *Asbestos*

*Asbestos Exposure: What It Means, What To Do.* Publication 86-1594, National Cancer Institute, 1985.

*Guidance for Controlling Asbestos-Containing Material in Buildings.* Environmental Protection Agency, 1985.

Loveys, Ralph A. "Asbestos: Two Troubling Aspects." *The New York Times*, October 2, 1988.

*Robson, Barbara. "Asbestos in Our Water Supply." US Magazine*, February 9, 1987.

*The Inside Story: A Guide to Indoor Air Quality.* United States Environmental Protection Agency, September 1988.

Winter, Ruth. *Cancer-Causing Agents.* New York: Crown Publishers, 1979.

## Chapter 13 / *Formaldehyde*

Dadd, Debra Lynn. *Nontoxic and Natural.* Los Angeles, CA: Jeremy P. Tarcher, 1984.

————*Nontoxic, Natural and Earthwise.* Los Angeles, CA: Jeremy P. Tarcher, 1990.

————*The Nontoxic Home.* Los Angeles, CA: Jeremy P. Tarcher, 1986.

"Toxic carpets and the alternatives." *The Earthwise Consumer,* Mid-spring 1990.

*The Inside Story: A Guide to Indoor Air Quality.* United States Environmental Protection Agency, September 1988.

*Urea-Formaldehyde Foam Insulation (UFFI): What is UFFI and what is wrong with it?* Public Citizen Health Research Group Publication 775.

Winter, Ruth. *Cancer-Causing Agents.* New York: Crown Publishers, 1979.

**Chapter 14 /    *Garbage***

"Appliances No One Wants." *The New York Times,* October 1, 1988.

Breen, Bill. "Burn It? Do Incinerators Convert Waste to Energy or Trash to Toxics?" *Garbage: The Practical Journal for the Environment,* March–April 1991.

Brown, Ken. "Victory for Clean Air." *Clean Water Action News,* Winter 1991.

Cahn, Robert, ed. *An Environmental Agenda for the Future.* Washington, DC: Island Press, 1985.

Cole, Henry S., PhD, and R. Collins. "Mercury Rising." *Clean Water Action News,* Winter 1991.

Collins, Clare. "A Town Gains Its Fame for What It Does With Its Garbage." *The New York Times,* May 15, 1988.

Collins, Robert. "Recycle First: Countering the Rush to Burn." *Clean Water Action News,* Winter 1989.

Dadd, Debra Lynn. *Nontoxic, Natural and Earthwise.* Los Angeles, CA: Jeremy P. Tarcher, 1990.

Egan, Timothy. "Curbside Pickup and Sludge Forests: Some Cities Make Recycling Work." *The New York Times,* October 24, 1988.

Freeman, Theresa. "Garbage Incineration: Beating Back the Ash Attack." *Everyone's Back Yard,* Vol. 6, No. 4, Winter 1988.

Fromm, Steven. "Questions Linger About the Safety of Burning Trash." *The Trenton Times,* July 1, 1988.

"The Greenkeeping Resource Center." *Greenkeeping,* July/August 1991.

Hang, Walter Liong-Ting. *Lessons from Europe: Waste Recycling Versus Incineration.* New York Public Interest Research Group, 1986.

Hinds, Michael de Courcy. 3Do Disposable Diapers Ever Go Away?" *The New York Times,* February 25, 1989.

Luoma, Jon R. "Cities Turn to a New Generation of Incinerators for Garbage." *The New York Times,* August 2, 1988.

Marinelli, Janet. "Garbage at the Grocery." *Garbage: The Practical Journal for the Environment,* September–October 1989.

Meier, Barry. "U.S. Advice on Trash Causes Uproar." *The New York Times,* January 28, 1991.

"No Spot is Too Remote for Seagoing Trash." *The New York Times,* July 16, 1991.

"Nontoxic Batteries." *East West*, July–August 1991.
"Pack It Right." *Nutrition Action Health Letter*, April 1990.
"Plagued by Packaging." New York Public Interest Research Group Agenda, Winter 1990.
Underwood, Joanna D., Allen Hershkowitz, and Maarten deKadt. *Garbage: Practices, Problems and Remedies*. New York: INFORM, 1988.
——"To Solve Trash Crisis: Recycle, Generate Less Waste." *Not Man Apart*, November 1988–January 1989.
"USA Snapshots: Wastewall, Coast to Coast." *USA Today*, June 24, 1991.
Wasson, John and Stephanie Pollack. "The Waste Land." *Science for the People*, November–December 1987.

### Chapter 15 / *Hazardous-Waste Sites*

Atwood, Sam. "Superfund: Boon or bust? Debate rages on." *USA Today*, April 22, 1991.
Brown, Michael H. "Love Canal Revisited." *Amicus Journal*, Summer 1988.
Cole, Henry S. and Bill Walsh. *Superfund 1987: Public Health Remains at Risk*. Clean Water Action Project, 1097.
Griffin, Melanie L. "The Legacy of Love Canal." *Sierra*, January–February 1988.
Hamilton, Robert A. "Dioxin-How Much is Too Much?" *The New York Times*, November 1, 1987.
"Hazardous Wastes: from Cradle to Grave." The State University of New Jersey Rutgers Environmental and Occupational Sciences Institute Infoletter, Spring 1990.
Hirschhorn, Joel S. "Preserving Our Environment: Preventing Hazardous Waste." *Science for the People*, September–October 1988.
Hoversten, Paul. "Some military bases will never be cleaned up." *USA Today*, July 5, 1991.
Reinganum, Charla B. and Walter L.T. Hang. "Toxic Wastelands: Environmental and Public Health Implications of Six New York City Municipal Landfills." New York Public Interest Research Group, 1983.
Resnikoff, Marvin. *Living Without Landfills*. New York: Radioactive Waste Campaign, 1988.
Schneider, Keith. "Squandering the Superfund." United States Public Interest Research Group Citizen Agenda, Fall 1988.

### Chapter 16 / *Indoor Pollution and Household Products*

Aveney, Rachel. *Children Beware: Art Supplies in the Classroom*. New York Public Interest Research Group and Center for Occupational Hazards, 1982.
*CBE Fact Sheet*. Chicago: Citizens for a Better Environment.
*Clean Water Action Project Consumer Guide to Toxic and Non-Toxic Household Products*. Clean Water Action, 1988.
Dadd, Debra Lynn. *Nontoxic and Natural*. Los Angeles, CA: Jeremy P. Tarcher, 1984.
Fossel, Peter. "SickHome Blues." *Harrowsmith Country Life*, September/October 1987.

Galvin, David and Sally Toteff. "Toxics on the Home Front." *Sierra,* September–October 1986.

Horowitz, Robert. "Does Danger Lurk in Your Attic?" *Public Citizen,* July–August 1991.

*Indoor Air Pollution Fact Sheet.* United States Environmental Protection Agency, June 1985.

Reuben, Carolyn. "Warning: Your Home May Be Hazardous To Your Health." *East West,* July 1989.

Rinzler, Carol Ann. *The Consumers Brand-Name Guide to Household Products.* New York: Lippincott and Crowell, 1980.

*Stepping Lightly on the Earth: Everyone's Guide to Toxics in the Home.* Greenpeace, 1988.

Taxel, Laura. "Color Me Safe: Nontoxic Art Supplies." *EastWest Natural Health,* May/June 1992.

*The Complete Book of Cancer Prevention.* Emmaus, PA: Rodale Press, 1988.

*The Inside Story: A Guide to Indoor Air Quality.* United States Environmental Protection Agency, September 1988.

*Toxics in the Home.* New Jersey Department of Environmental Protection, Division of Hazardous Waste Management, Hazardous Waste Advisement Program.

**Chapter 17 /** *Lead*

Boling, Rick. "Heavy Metal." *Harrowsmith,* Vol. 1, No. 6, November–December 1986.

Burros, Marion. "Eating Well: Recalls of Ceramic Ware That Release High Levels of Lead May Be the Tip of the Iceberg." *The New York Times,* July 13, 1988.

"Death From Lead Exposure Prompts Call for Yearly Tests." *The New York Times,* March 29, 1991.

French, Howard W. "High Lead Level Found in Water in Many Areas." *The New York Times,* November 17, 1988.

French, Janet Beighle. "Kit tests toxicity of lead in dishes." *The Plain Dealer,* December 2, 1987.

Goode, Erica E. "Putting the Lid on Dangerous Dinnerware." *U.S. News and World Report,* August 10, 1987.

*Lead and Your Drinking Water.* United States Environmental Protection Agency, April 1987.

Lecos, Chris W. "Pretty Poison: Lead and Ceramic Ware." *FDA Consumer,* July–August 1987.

Mead, Nathaniel. "Lead Alert: An Age-Old Problem May Be Affecting Your Child." *East West Magazine,* July–August 1991.

Ochs, Ridgely. "Looking Out for Lead in Pottery." *Newsday,* January 15, 1987.

"New Data Show Continued Risk of Lead Poisoning." *The New York Times,* August 20, 1988.

Taxel, Laura. "Color Me Safe: Nontoxic Art Supplies." *EastWest Natural Health,* May/June 1992.

The Inside Story: A Guide to Indoor Air Quality. United States Environmental Protection Agency, September 1988.

Waldman, Steven. "Lead and Your Kids." *Newsweek*, July 15, 1991.

Weinhouse, Beth. "Lead Pottery Warning." *Ladies Home Journal*, December 1987.

Weisskopf, Michael. "Don't Drink the Water and Don't Lick the Plate." *The Washington Post*, January 12, 1987.

————"Lead Astray: The Poisoning of America." *Discover*, December 1987.

Winter, Ruth. *Cancer-Causing Agents*. New York: Crown Publishers, 1979.

### Chapter 18 / *Nuclear Waste*

Berger, Dr. Jonathan, ed. *Radiation Monitoring System for Nuclear Power Plants*. Three Mile Island Public Health Fund, December 1987.

Cahn, Robert, ed. *An Environmental Agenda for the Future*. Washington, DC: Island Press, 1985.

Carpenter, Tom. "America's Deadly Defense: A Double-Edged Sword." *Radioactive Waste Campaign (RWC) Waste Paper*, Spring 1988.

"CCRI Sponsors New Childhood Cancer Study." The Childhood Cancer Research Institute, January 1991.

Clapp, Richard, ScD. "Two New Studies on Cancers Near Nuclear Facilities." The Childhood Cancer Research Institute, January 1991.

Coyle, Dan et al. *Deadly Defense: Military Radioactive Landfills*. New York: Radioactive Waste Campaign, 1988.

Davis, Joseph A. "The Wasting of Nevada." *Sierra*, July–August 1988.

DeerInWater, Jessie. "Nuclear Waste Used as Fertilizer in Oklahoma." *Radioactive Waste Campaign (RWC) Waste Paper*, Fall 1988.

Fazzino, Jean. "Crisis at the Nuclear Bomb Plants: Weapons Plants Coming Apart at Seams." *Radioactive Waste Campaign (RWC) Waste Paper*, Winter 1988–89.

Franklin, Ben A. "Defective Bolts Found in Half of Nuclear Reactors." *The New York Times*, June 19, 1988.

Hoversten, Paul. "Some military bases will never be cleaned up." *USA Today*, July 5, 1991.

Kneale, G.W. and A. M. Stewart. "Childhood Cancers in the UK and their Relation to Background Radiation." *Radiation and Health*, 1987.

Maize, Ken. "DOE Weapons Program: 'They Lied to Us.'" *Not Man Apart*, November 1988–January 1989.

Murphy, Joan. "The Battle Over Nuclear America." *Public Citizen*, May–June 1990.

Quigley, Diane. "A Summary of Occupational Studies on Cancer Mortality of Nuclear Workers." The Childhood Cancer Research Institute, October 1991.

"Report calls military nations worst polluters." *The New York Times*, March 17, 1991.

Resnikoff, Marvin. "Nuclear Wastes—The Myths and the Realities." *Sierra*, July–August 1980.

————*Radioactive Waste Campaign: The First Ten Years*. New York: Radioactive Waste Campaign, 1988.

Roberts, Leslie. "British Radiation Study Throws Experts intoTizzy." *Science*, April 1990.

Schneider, Keith. " Accidents at a U.S. Nuclear Plant Were Kept Secret Up To 31 Years." *The New York Times*, September 30, 1989.

————"Leaking Mine Threatens A Waste Storage Plan." *The New York Times*, February 1, 1988.

————"U.S. May Yield Health Data on Nuclear Weapons Workers." *The New York Times*, October 28, 1988.

————"U.S. Studies Health Problems Near Weapons Plants." *The New York Times*, October 17, 1988.

————"Wide Threat Seen in Contamination at Nuclear Plants." *The New York Times*, December 7, 1988.

Stine, Annie. "Scarcely Watched Trains." *Sierra*, March–April 1988.

Sullivan, Walter. "Three Mile Island Cleanup Uncovers New Details." *The New York Times*, January 26, 1988.

Tyson, Rae. "Report says toxic spills on increase." *USA Today*, July 25, 1991.

Wald, Matthew L. "Wider Peril Seen in Northwest from Bomb Making." *The New York Times*, March 28, 1991.

Warner, Gale. "Low-Level Lowdown." *Sierra*, July–August 1985.

Winchester, Ellen. "Nuclear Wastes." *Sierra*, July–August 1979.

## Chapter 19 /  *Outdoor Hazards*

Babbitt, Bruce. "Nowhere to Hide." *Amicus Journal*, Fall 1988.

Begley, Sharon, Mark Miller, and Mary Hager. "The Endless Summer?" *Newsweek*, July 11, 1988.

Broad, William J. "Scientists Dream Up Bold Remedies for Ailing Atmosphere." *The New York Times*, August 16, 1988.

Brody, Jane E. "Determining Why Smog Can Be Deadly." *The New York Times*, February 21, 1989.

Browne, Malcolm W. "New Tactics Emerge in Struggle Against Smog." *The New York Times*, February 21, 1989.

Cahn, Robert, ed. *An Environmental Agenda for the Future*. Washington, DC: Island Press, 1985.

Crossette, Linda B. "Manufacturers Develop Better Skin Products." *Journal of the National Cancer Institute*, June 5, 1991.

Elias, Marilyn. "Vitamin E oil may help curb skin cancer." *USA Today*, May 30, 1991.

————"Early years count most in skin cancer risk." *USA Today*, November 20, 1991.

Goldfarb, Bruce. "In summertime, safety precautions make the living easy." *USA Today*, May 30, 1991.

"Group Says EPA needs to expand unhealthy air list." *USA Today*, July 26, 1991.

Hanson, Beth. "The Ultraviolet Zone." *Amicus Journal*, Summer 1991.

"Helter Swelter: Earth's Climate Goes Awry." *Sierra*, January–February 1988.

"Home Stretch to Clean Air." United States Public Interest Research Group Citizen Agenda, Summer 1988.

Kanamine, Linda. "Coalition: EPA not cleaning up smog." *USA Today*, July 26, 1991.

Kolbert, Elizabeth. "Acid Rain Imperils Adirondack Fish." *The New York Times*, July 7, 1988.

LaBastille, Anne. "The International Acid Test." *Sierra*, May–June 1986.

Luoma, Jon R. "Damaged Wildlife Shows Pollution Still Plagues Great Lakes." *The New York Times*, January 12, 1988.

Lyman, Francesca. "As the Ozone Thins, the Plot Thickens." *Amicus Journal*, Summer 1991.

Mead, Nathaniel. "Oh Those Hazy Days of Summer." *East West*, June 1991.

Milne, Anthony. *Our Drowning World: Population, Pollution and Future Weather*. Garden City Park, NY: Prism Press, 1989.

Mintz, Penny. "CFCs: Just Say No." *Amicus Journal*, Summer 1991.

"Ozone depletion faster than thought." *USA Today*, May 5, 1991.

Schneider, Keith. "Ozone Depletion Harming Sea Life." *The New York Times*, November 16, 1991.

Shabecoff, Philip. "Acid Rain is Called Peril for Sea Life on Atlantic Coast." *The New York Times*, April 25, 1988.

————"Global Warming: Experts Ponder Bewildering Feedback Effects." *The New York Times*, January 17, 1989.

————"Health Risk from Smog is Growing, Official Says." *The New York Times*, March 1, 1988.

————"Major Greenhouse Impact is Unavoidable, Experts Say." *The New York Times*, July 19, 1988.

————"U.S. Calls Poisoning of Air Far Worse Than Expected and Threat to Public." *The New York Times*, March 23, 1989.

Stevens, William K. "Ozone Layer Thinner, but Forces Are in Place for Slow Improvement." *The New York Times*, April 9, 1991.

————"Urgent Steps Urged on Warming Threat." *The New York Times*, April 11, 1991.

Sullivan, Scott. "Nature's Revenge." *Newsweek*, March 2, 1987.

Wald, Matthew L. "Fighting the Greenhouse Effect." *The New York Times*, August 28, 1988.

Whipple, Dan. "King Copper's Acid Rain." *Sierra*, March–April, 1985.

**Chapter 20 /** *Pesticides in the Home and Yard*

*A Citizen's Guide to Pesticides*. United States Environmental Protection Agency, September 1987.

"Armoring Against Mosquitoes.L *East West*, June 1991.

Allen, Frank Edward. "One Man's Suffering Spurs Doctors to Probe Pesticide-Drug Link." *The Wall Street Journal*, October 14, 1991.

Dadd, Debra Lynn. *Nontoxic and Natural*. Los Angeles, CA: Jeremy P. Tarcher, 1984.

————*Nontoxic, Natural and Earthwise*. Los Angeles, CA: Jeremy P. Tarcher, 1990.

————*The NonToxic Home.* Los Angeles, CA: Jeremy P. Tarcher, 1986.
"Insect repellents Containing Ethyl Hexanediol." Washington, DC: Public
    Citizen Health Research Group Health Letter, November 1991.
"Mailbasket." *The Earthwise Consumer,* Late Winter–Early Spring 1991.
Meier, Barry. "Battle of the Bugs, Is Stronger Better?" *The New York Times,*
    July 20, 1991.
*Pesticides and You: Chemical Watch.* National Campaign Against the Misuse
    of Pesticides, March 1989.
*Pesticide Safety.* Washington, DC: National Campaign Against the Misuse
    of Pesticides, 1988.
Potter, Jerry. "LPGA learns realities of breast cancer." *USA Today,* Novem-
    ber 7, 1991.
Reuben, Carolyn. "Warning: Your Home May Be Hazardous To Your
    Health." *East West,* July 1989.
Schneider, Keith. "Senate Panel Says Lawn Chemicals Harm Many." *The
    New York Times,* May 10, 1991.
*Stepping Lightly on the Earth: Everyone's Guide to Toxics in the Home.* Wash-
    ington, DC: Greenpeace, 1988.
*The Complete Book of Cancer Prevention.* Emmaus, PA: Rodale Press, 1988.
"Weed Killer May Hold Cancer Risk." *New York Newsday,* September 4,
    1991.

### Chapter 21 /    *Pet Products*

Holmes, Hannah. "Run, Spot, Run!" *Garbage: A Practical Journal for the
    Environment,* July–August 1991.
"Lawn Herbicide Called Cancer Risk to Dogs." *The New York Times,*
    September 4, 1991.
Manning, Anita. "Organic pet products gain a paw-hold." *USA Today,*
    July 22, 1991.
Marder, Amy, VMD. "Natural Flea and Tick Control." *Prevention,* July
    1991.
Snider, Mike. "Weedkiller threat to dogs." *USA Today,* September 4, 1991.

### Chapter 22 /    *Radiation in the Home*

Altman, Lawrence K. "Some Who Use VDTs Miscarried, Study Says." *The
    New York Times,* June 5, 1988.
Becker, Robert O., MD. *Cross Currents: The Promise of Electromedicine, the
    Perils of Electropollution.* Los Angeles, CA: Jeremy P. Tarcher, 1990.
Blakeslee, Sandra. "Electromagnetic Fields are Being Scrutinized for
    Linkage to Cancer." *The New York Times,* April 2, 1991.
Brodeur, Paul. "Radiation in Daily Life." *US Magazine,* December 1, 1986.
————*Currents of Death: Power Lines, Computer Terminals, and the Attempt
    to Cover Up Their Threat to Your Health.* New York: Simon & Schuster,
    1990.
Dadd, Debra Lynn. *The Nontoxic Home.* Los Angeles, CA: Jeremy P.
    Tarcher, 1986.
————*Nontoxic, Natural and Earthwise.* Los Angeles, CA: Jeremy P.
    Tarcher, 1990.

Davidoff, Linda Lee. "Multiple Chemical Sensitivities." *Amicus Journal,* Vol. 11, No. 1, Winter 1989.

"Electromagnetic fields—What You Can Do to Protect Yourself From This Invisible Danger." *The Earthwise Consumer,* Late Summer/Early Autumn 1990.

Good, Clint and Debra Lynn Dadd. "Buying the Healthful House." *East West,* July 1989.

"How Healthful is Your Home?" *East West,* July 1989.

"Kids Wired for Cancer." *East West,* July–August 1991.

Lechter, George M. *Facts on Electromagnetic Radiation.* Needham, MA: Safe Technologies Corporation, 1991.

Lewin, Tamar. "Miscarriages at USA Today Are Under Review." *The New York Times,* December 10, 1988.

Mayell, Mark. "Around the Home: Smoke Detectors, the Non-Nuclear Alternative." *East West,* April 1990.

Monte, Tom. "In Search of the Healthful House." *East West,* July 1989.

"NCI and CCSG Examine the Role of Magnetic Fields in Childhood Leukemia." *Journal of the National Cancer Institute,* February 7, 1990.

Schechter, Steven R. with T. Monte. *Fighting Radiation with Foods, Herbs and Vitamins.* Brookline, MA: East West Health Books, 1988.

"Study Links VDTs to Miscarriages." *Science for the People,* September–October 1988.

Skiba, Joy Taylor. "Get the Most from a Microwave." *Parade Magazine,* October 25, 1987.

"Tungsten-Halogen Bulbs May Pose a Hazard." *The New York Times,* July 30, 1991.

**Chapter 23 /  *Radon***

*A Citizen's Guide to Radon: What It Is and What To Do About It.* United States Environmental Protection Agency, August 1986.

Adkins, Jason B. and Daniel H. Pink. "Radon: What You Don't Know Can Hurt You." *Public Citizen,* Vol. 7, No. 3, April 1987.

Blot, W. et al. "Indoor Radon and Lung Cancer." *Journal of the National Cancer Institute,* June 20, 1990.

"Experts Debate Radon Risk." *Journal of the National Cancer Institute,* June 19, 1991.

Friend, Tim. "Kits may overstate radon risk." *USA Today,* March 29, 1991.

Johnson, Kirk. " Radon Primer." *East West,* November 1987.

LaFavore, Michael. *Radon: The Invisible Threat.* Emmaus, PA: Rodale Press, 1987.

Leary, Warren E. "13,000 Deaths a Year Indicated by Science Academy Radon Study." *The New York Times,* January 6, 1988.

Mead, Nathaniel. "The Riddle of Radon." *East West,* July 1990.

*Radon Reduction Methods: A Homeowner's Guide.* United States Environmental Protection Agency, 1986.

"Radon: Where It Originates and What Can Be Done About It." *The New York Times,* September 13, 1988.

Shabecoff, Philip. *"Major Radon Peril is Declared by U.S. in Call for Tests."* The
    *New York Times,* September 13, 1988.
The Inside Story: A Guide to Indoor Air Quality. United States Environ-
    mental Protection Agency, September 1988.

**Chapter 24 /**    *Stoves, Heaters, and Fireplaces*

Dadd, Debra Lynn. *Nontoxic and Natural.* Los Angeles, CA: Jeremy P.
    Tarcher, 1984.
————*Nontoxic, Natural and Earthwise.* Los Angeles, CA: Jeremy P.
    Tarcher, 1990.
————*The Nontoxic Home.* Los Angeles, CA: Jeremy P. Tarcher, 1986.
"Now They Tell Us!" *Newsweek,* April 1, 1991.
The Inside Story: A Guide to Indoor Air Quality. United States Environ-
    mental Protection Agency, September 1988.

**Chapter 25 /**    *Water*

"A Strategy to Protect Groundwater." *Clean Water Action News,* Summer
    1987.
Brody, Jane E. "Personal Health: As Contamination of Surface and Under-
    ground Water Rises, How Safe is the Water We Drink?" *The New York
    Times,* October 6, 1988.
Carney, Leo H. "Coastal Pollution: No Quick Remedy Seen." *The New York
    Times,* August 28, 1988.
Conacher, Duff and Associates. *Troubled Waters on Tap: Organic Chemicals
    in Public Drinking Water Systems and the Failure of Regulation.* Washing-
    ton, DC: Center for the Study of Responsive Law, January 1988.
Dadd, Debra Lynn. "Buyers Guide to Water Purification Devices." *Every-
    thing Natural,* 1987.
————*Nontoxic and Natural.* Los Angeles, CA: Jeremy P. Tarcher, 1984.
Draper, Eric. "Ground Water Protection." *Clean Water Action News,* Fall
    1987.
"Drinking Water." *Buyers Market,* Vol. 3, No. 1, March 1987.
*Eating Clean: Overcoming Food Hazards.* Washington, DC: Center for the
    Study of Responsive Law, 1988.
Guernsey, Paul. "Contaminants Seeping Into Ground Water Supplies."
    *The New York Times,* January 17, 1988.
"Home Water Treatment Systems: Another Alternative." *Buyers Market,*
    Vol.13, No. 1, March 1987.
Konner, Bernice. "On the Water Front: The Boom in Bottled Waters." *The
    New York Times,* May 9, 1988.
Lefferts, Lisa Y. and Stephen B. Schmidt. "Water: Safe to Swallow?"
    *Nutrition Action Health Letter,* November 1988.
McDonald, Jacqueline. "Home Water Purifiers: How to Make a Rational
    Purchase." *Garbage, The Practical Journal for the Environment.* March–
    April 1991.
"NRDC's campaign for clean water." Washington, DC: *Natural Resources
    Defense Council Newsline,* July 1991.

Schmidt, William E. "Iowans Struggle Against Rising Water Pollution." *The New York Times*, November 22, 1987.
Shabecoff, Philip. "Pollution is Blamed for Killing Whales in St. Lawrence." *The New York Times*, January 12, 1988.
Stanfield, Rochelle L. "Some Scientists See Key to Water Pollution in Thin Surface Layer." *The New York Times*, June 21, 1988.
————"Treatment of Sewage is Seen as Insufficient to Protect Water." *The New York Times*, September 13, 1988.
Tunley, Roul. "Is Your Water Safe?" *Readers' Digest*, November 1986.
"12 Tips for Tap Water Cleanup." *Prevention*, June 1989.
Wilson, Reid. *Toxics on Tap*. Washington, DC: United States Public Information Research Group, May 1986.

## Chapter 26 /   X-Rays

Johnsrud, Judith H., PhD. "On the Trail of Childhood Cancers." *EastWest*, November 1987.
"Ten Tests That Can Save your Life From the American College of Radiology." *Prevention*, April 1988.
*The Complete Book of Cancer Prevention*. Emmaus, PA: Rodale Press, 1988.
Schottenfeld, David, MD, and Joseph F. Fraumeni, Jr., MD. *Cancer Epidemiology and Prevention*. Philadelphia, PA: W.B. Saunders Company, 1982.

## Chapter 27 /   AIDS

Altman, Lawrence K. "Who's Stricken and How: AIDS Pattern is Shifting." *The New York Times*, February 5, 1989.
————"Gains Cited on AIDS, But Urgency Remains." *The New York Times*, June 25, 1991.
"Can You Rely on Condoms?" *Consumer Reports*, March 1989.
DePalma, Anthony. "No Conclusion on Ways Dentist Passed AIDS." *The New York Times*, June 26, 1991.
*Facts About AIDS*. United States Public Health Service, Centers for Disease Control.
*How You Won't Get AIDS*. United States Public Health Service, Centers for Disease Control.
Koop, C. Everett, MD. "Surgeon General's Report on Acquired Immune Deficiency Syndrome." United States Department of Health and Human Services, 1988.
Melton, George and W. Garcia. "Beyond AIDS: A journey into healing." *USA Today*, June 24, 1991.
Moffatt, Betty Clare, J. Spiegel, S. Parrish, and M. Helquist, eds. *AIDS: A Self-Care Manual*. Santa Monica, CA: IBS Press, 1988.
Puente, Maria and K. Painter. "Report: AIDS dentist lied to save practice." *USA Today*, June 24, 1991.
"Safe and Natural Sex: Protecting Yourself from AIDS." *Everything Natural*, May–June 1987.

Sattar, Syed A. and V.S. Springthorpe. "Survival and Disinfectant Activation of the Human Immunodeficiency Virus: A Critical Review." *Reviews of Infectious Diseases,* May–June 1991.
"What You Should Know About AIDS." United States Public Health Service, Centers for Disease Control.

### Chapter 28 /   Cosmetics and Personal-Care Products

*Being Beautiful.* Washington, DC: Center for the Study of Responsive Law, 1986.
Brody, Jane E. "Personal Health." *The New York Times,* September 19, 1984.
Dadd, Debra Lynn. *Nontoxic and Natural.* Los Angeles, CA: Jeremy P. Tarcher, 1984.
"Estrogens in Cosmetics." *The Medical Letter,* June 21, 1985.
Morrison, Margaret. *Cosmetics: The Substance Beneath the Form.* United States Department of Health, Education and Welfare, Food and Drug Administration, Publication (FDA) 78-5007, 1979.
Piver, M. Steven et al. "Epidemiology and etiology of ovarian cancer." *Seminars in Oncology,* June 1991.
Report to the Congress of the United States by the Comptroller General. General Accounting Office, August 1988.
*The Complete Book of Cancer Prevention.* Emmaus, PA: Rodale Press, 1988.
Winter, Ruth. *A Consumer's Dictionary of Cosmetic Ingredients.* New York: Crown Publishers, 1984.
———*Cancer-Causing Agents.* New York: Crown Publishers, 1979.

### Chapter 29 /   Estrogen and Birth Control Pills

Carper, Jean. *The Food Pharmacy.* New York: Bantam Books, 1988.
Dardick, Geeta. "Breast Self Exam: A New Program Makes Detection Easier." *East West,* July–August 1991.
Heinerman, John. *Encyclopedia of Fruits, Vegetables, and Herbs.* West Nyack, NY: Parker Publishing, 1988.
Kolata, Gina. "New Data on the Pill Find Breast Cancer as a Possible Link." *The New York Times,* May 5, 1989.
Lublin, Joann S. "Young Women on Pill May Run a Greater Risk of Breast Cancer." *The Wall Street Journal,* May 5, 1989.
"New British Study Links Pill and Breast Cancer." *National Alliance of Breast Cancer Organizations (NABCO) News III* (3):3, July 1989.
Okie, Susan and S. Rovner. "Breast Cancer and the Pill: What Women Need to Know." *The Washington Post,* January 10, 1989.
"Reducing the Risk of Breast Cancer." *Nutrition Action Health Letter,* March 1987.
"Swedish Studies Link Hormone Use to Higher Breast Cancer Risk." *Journal of the National Cancer Institute,* August 16, 1989.
*The Complete Book of Cancer Prevention.* Emmaus, PA: Rodale Press, 1988.
Wolfe, Sidney. "New Evidence that Menopausal Estrogens Cause Breast Cancer." *Public Citizen Health Research Group Health Letter,* June 1991.

**Chapter 30 /** *Lack of Exercise*

Barone, Jeanine. "Can Diet Protect Your Immune System?" *Nutrition Action Health Letter*, August 1988.

Benjamin, Harold H., PhD. *From Victim to Victor*. New York: Bantam Doubleday Dell Publishing Group, 1987.

Cooper, Kenneth. *The Aerobic Program for Total Well-Being: Exercise, Diet, Emotional Balance*. New York: M. Evans & Company, 1982.

Hoffman, S.A. and K.E. Paschikis et al. "The Influence of Exercise on the Growth of Transplanted Rat Tumors." *Cancer Patient* Vol. 22, pp. 597–99, 1962.

Marchetti, Albert, MD. *Beating the Odds*. Chicago: Contemporary Books, 1988.

Selye, Hans. *The Stress of Life*. New York: McGraw-Hill, 1958.

Simonton, Stephanie Matthews, O. Carl Simonton, MD, and James L. Creighton. *Getting Well Again*. New York: Bantam Books, 1978.

Snider, Mike. "Exercise workouts may lessen cancer risk." *USA Today*, September 5, 1991.

*The Complete Book of Cancer Prevention*. Emmaus, PA: Rodale Press, 1988.

Walker, Morton. *Jumping for Health*. Garden City Park, NY: Avery Publishing Group, 1989.

Whittemore, A.S. et al. "Diet, physical acticity and colorectal cancer among Chinese in North America and China." *Journal of the National Cancer Institute*, June 6, 1990.

**Chapter 31 /** *Obesity*

Brody, Jane E. "Personal Health: The fat to fear, the experts say, is around the middle." *The New York Times*, November 20, 1991.

Jacobson, Michael F., PhD. *The Complete Eater's Digest and Nutrition Scoreboard*. Garden City, NY: Anchor Press/Doubleday, 1985.

Marchetti, Albert, MD. *Beating the Odds*. Chicago: Contemporary Books, 1988.

*Nutrition and Your Health: Dietary Guidelines for Americans*. United States Department of Agriculture and United States Department of Health and Human Services, 2nd Edition, 1985.

Pi-Sunyer, F. Xavier. "Health Implications of Obesity." *American Journal of Clinical Nutrition*, June 1991.

*The Complete Book of Cancer Prevention*. Emmaus, PA: Rodale Press, 1988.

Webb, Denise. "Eating Well: Obesity is hazardous; so is a failed diet." *The New York Times*, November 20, 1991.

**Chapter 32 /** *Silicone Implants*

"Background Information on the Possible Health Risks of Silicone Breast Implants." Food and Drug Administration, February 8, 1991.

Blakeslee, Sandra. "Breast Implant Maker Asks Doctors Not to Use Device Linked to Cancer." *The New York Times*, April 18, 1991.

"Breast Reconstruction: Risks and Benefits." *NABCO News*, July 1991.

"Doctors Urged to be Frank on Breast Implant Risks." *The New York Times,* August 1, 1991.

"$4 Million Awarded in Breast-Implant Case." *The New York Times,* March 24, 1991.

Hilts, Philip J. "Scientists Tie Breast Implants to Cancer." *The New York Times,* April 14, 1991.

————"Vigilance is Called Essential For Women With Implants." *The New York Times,* January 8, 1992.

Painter, Kim. "FDA: Stop silicone breast implants." *USA Today,* January 7, 1992.

"Silicone Gel Implants Cause Cancer." Washington, DC: Public Citizen Health Research Group Health Letter, December 1988.

"Update on Silicone Breast Implants." *NABCO News,* July 1991.

## Chapter 33 / *Smoking: Active and Passive*

Bauman, Karl E., R.L. Flewlling, and J. LaPrelle. "Parental Smoking and Cognitive Performance of Children." *Health Psychology,* October 1991.

Brody, Jane E. "New Study Strongly Links Passive Smoking and Cancer." *The New York Times,* January 8, 1992.

*Cancer Facts and Figures.* American Cancer Society, 1991.

"Cigarette smoking and the risk of breast cancer." *American Journal of Epidemiology,* September 1990.

*Clearing the Air: A Guide to Quitting Smoking.* National Cancer Institute Publication 85-1647, 1986.

*Clearing the Air: How to Quit Smoking and Quit for Keeps.* National Cancer Institute, 1987.

Farrow, D.C. et al. "Risk of pancreatic cancer in relation to medical history and the use of tobacco, alcohol and coffee." *International Journal of Cancer,* May 1990.

Friend, Tim. "Smokers' kids run twice the health risk." *USA Today,* June 18, 1991.

————"Smoking, a colon cancer risk." July 3, 1991.

"Good News for Former Smokers from Surgeon General Novello." *Journal of the National Cancer Institute,* December 5, 1990.

Herrera, R. et al. "Invasive cervical cancer and smoking in Latin America." *Journal of the National Cancer Institute,* February 1, 1989.

Hilts, Philip J. "High Death Toll Seen from Passive Smoking." *The New York Times,* May 10, 1991.

LaVecchia, C. et al. "Smoking and renal cell carcinoma." *Cancer Research,* September 1990.

Licciardone, J.C. et al. "Cigarette smoking and alcohol in the aetiology of uterine and cervical cancer." *International Journal of Epidemiology,* September 1989.

Namura, A. et al. "Smoking, alcohol and hair dye use in cancer of lower urinary tract." *American Journal of Epidemiology,* June 1990.

"Passive Smoking: Exposure Occurs on Commercial Flights." *Journal of the National Cancer Institute,* March 15, 1989.

"Research Studies Tobacco-Breast Cancer Link." *The New York Times,* September 27, 1988.

Sandler, Dale P., PhD., et al. "Deaths from all causes in nonsmokers who lived with smokers." *American Journal of Epidemiology,* October 4, 1988.

"Secondhand Smoke Assailed in Report." *The New York Times,* May 30, 1991.

"Smoking Cessation: The Best Ways to Kick the Deadliest, Most Expensive Addiction." Public Citizen Health Research Group Health Letter, Vol. 4, No. 10, October 1988.

"Smokeless Tobacco Linked to Oral Lesions." *The New York Times,* January 17, 1989.

"Smoking Hastens Facial Wrinkles, Study Finds." *The New York Times,* July 2, 1991.

Snider, Mike. "Passive smoke's harmful effects can't be gauged." *USA Today,* April 19, 1991.

*The Complete Book of Cancer Prevention.* Emmaus, PA: Rodale Press, 1988.

*The Merck Manual of Diagnosis and Therapy,* 15th Edition, Merck & Company, 1987.

Tolchin, Martin. "Surgeon General Asserts Smoking is an Addiction." *The New York Times,* May 17, 1988.

Winkelstein, W., Jr. "Smoking and cervical cancer: current status." *American Journal of Epidemiology,* June 1990.

## Chapter 34 / *Stress*

Achterberg, Jeanne. *Imagery in Healing.* Boston: Shambhala Publications, 1985.

Benjamin, Harold H., PhD. *From Victim to Victor.* New York: Bantam Doubleday Dell Publishing Group, 1987.

Benson, Herbert. *The Relaxation Response.* New York: William Morrow & Company, 1975.

Borysenko, Joan. *Minding the Body, Mending the Mind.* Reading, MA: Addison-Wesley Publishing Company, 1987.

"Can an Immune Response be Conditioned?" *Journal of the National Cancer Institute,* October 3, 1990.

Cousins, Norman. *Anatomy of an Illness as Perceived by the Patient: Reflections on Healing and Regeneration.* New York: W.W. Norton & Company, 1979.

———"Belief Becomes Biology." *Advances,* Vol. 6, No. 3, Fall 1989.

*Diagnostic and Statistical Manual of Mental Disorders.* Third Edition, The American Psychological Association, 1987 (rev).

Gawler, Ian, Dr. *Peace of Mind: How You Can Learn to Meditate and Use the Power of Your Mind.* Garden City Park, NY: Avery Publishing Group, 1989.

Goleman, Daniel. "Researchers Find That Optimism Helps the Body's Defense System." *The New York Times,* April 20, 1989.

Hornig Rohan, Mady, MD. "Abstracts of Studies Recently Published." *Advances: Journal of Mind-Body Health,* Summer 1991.

Johnson, Mark. *The Body in the Mind.* University of Chicago, 1989.
LeShan, Lawrence. *Cancer as a Turning Point.* New York: E.P. Dutton, 1989.
Marchetti, Albert, MD. *Beating the Odds.* Chicago: Contemporary Books, 1988.
"Meditators Need Less Medical Care." *East West,* July 1989.
Orme-Johnson, David Dr. *Psychosomatic Medicine,* Vol. 49, No. 5, 1989.
Pelletier, Kenneth. *Mind as Healer, Mind as Slayer.* New York: Dell Publishing Company, 1977.
"Psychoneuro Immunology: Can the Brain and the Immune System Communicate?" *Journal of the National Cancer Institute,* May 2, 1990.
Selye, Hans. *The Stress of Life.* New York: McGraw-Hill, 1956.
Siegel, Bernie, MD. *Love, Medicine and Miracles.* New York: Harper and Row, 1986.
———*Peace, Love and Healing.* New York: Harper and Row, 1989.
Simonton, Stephanie Mathews, O. Carl Simonton, and James L. Creighton. *Getting Well Again.* New York: Bantam Books, 1978.
"Stanford University Cancer Study Yields Surprising Results." *Foundation for Advancement in Cancer Therapy News,* March 1991.
Whelan, Jeremy. "Conference: Cancer and the mind." *Lancet,* February 24, 1990.
Zarrow, Susan and G. McVeish. "Hormones from Hell." *Prevention,* June 1991.

**Chapter 35 /  Workplace Hazards**

"Caution: An Ill Wind May Be Blowing in Your Office, Warns Building Doctor Gray Robertson." *People,* February 2, 1989.
*Communities and Workers Right to Know.* Washington, DC: United States Public Citizen Health Research Group, March 15, 1985.
Gotsch, Audrey R., Michelle Demak, and Amy Erhardt. "Environmental and Occupational Health Risks: A Model Information Program." *New Jersey Medicine,* Vol. 83, No. 7, July 1986.
*The Inside Story: A Guide to Indoor Air Quality.* United States Environmental Protection Agency, September 1991.
McCain, Mark. "It Pays to Hire Experts to Look for Contamination." *The New York Times,* October 25, 1987.
Milbank, Dana. "Link is Found Between Bladder Cancer and Two Chemicals Used in Industry." *Wall Street Journal,* April 3, 1991.
"Offices are harming millions of workers." *USA Today,* May 29, 1991.
Perkins, Jimmy L., PhD, and James D. Kimbrough, MSPH. "Formaldehyde Exposure in a Gross Anatomy Laboratory." *Journal of Occupational Medicine,* Vol. 27, No. 11, November 1985.
*Public Citizen Health Research Group Report on NIOSH Studies Showing Increased Worker Health Risks.* Public Citizen Health Research Group, January 23, 1985.
Schottenfeld, David, MD, and Joseph F. Fraumeni, Jr., MD. *Cancer Epidemiology and Prevention.* Philadelphia, PA: W.B. Saunders Company, 1982.

# INDEX